3RD EDITION

HEALTH MATTERS

ENGLISCH FÜR MEDIZINISCHE FACHANGESTELLTE

von
Ian Wood

sowie
Manfred Thönicke

unter Mitarbeit von
der Verlagsredaktion

Cornelsen

HEALTH MATTERS

Verfasser: Ian Wood, Linton, Großbritannien
Verfasser KMK-Seiten: Manfred Thönicke, Hamburg
Beraterin: Maren Stecker-Gössling, Duisburg
Projektleitung: Shaunessy Ashdown
Redaktionelle Mitarbeit: Jim Austin, Christine House, Oliver Busch (Wörterverzeichnisse)
Bildredaktion: Franziska Becker
Gesamtgestaltung und technische Umsetzung: vitaledesign, Berlin
Titelfoto: Fotolia/gamjai
Illustrationen: Oxford Designers & Illustrators

Erhältlich sind auch:
E-Book
ISBN 978-3-06-451420-1
Handreichungen für den Unterricht mit Audio-CD und Online-Zusatzmaterialien
ISBN 978-3-06-4514218

www.cornelsen.de

1. Auflage, 7. Druck 2026

Alle Drucke dieser Auflage sind inhaltlich unverändert und können im Unterricht nebeneinander verwendet werden.

Druck: Drukarnia Dimograf Sp. z o.o., Bielsko-Biała

ISBN 978-3-06-451420-1

Vorwort

Health Matters 3rd edition ist eine Neubearbeitung des bewährten Lehrwerks *Health Matters* für medizinische Fachangestellte für den Berufsschulunterricht und wurde aktualisiert und neu gestaltet.

Das einbändige Lehrwerk setzt Englischkenntnisse voraus, die dem Niveau A2 des Europäischen Referenzrahmens *(Common European Framework of Reference)* entsprechen. In der Rubrik *Extra Material* ist für Lernende mit fortgeschrittenen Englischkenntnissen anspruchsvollerer Lernstoff auf dem Niveau B1 enthalten. So wird eine kontinuierliche und differenzierte Förderung aller Zielgruppen gewährleistet und der Heterogenität der Auszubildenden Rechnung getragen.

Health Matters 3rd edition enthält 10 Units, in denen handlungsorientiert alltägliche berufstypische Situationen und aktuelle Themen aus unterschiedlichen Bereichen einer Arztpraxis und auch im Klinikbereich aufgegriffen werden. Landeskundliche Informationen über Großbritannien und die USA werden ebenfalls vermittelt. Der Schwerpunkt liegt auf dem dialogischen Austausch in typischen Berufssituationen. Dabei werden die kommunikativen, sprachlichen Kompetenzen anhand zahlreicher Hörverständnis- und Sprechübungen, die von rein funktionalen Dialogen bis zu freien Diskussionen reichen, geschult. Neu sind in diesem Zusammenhang Aufgabenstellungen, die gezielt die Kommunikation zwischen medizinischen Fachangestellten und Patienten/Patientinnen in berufstypischen Alltagsituationen fördern.

Anhand motivierender Aufgaben werden Hemmungen, sich in der Fremdsprache auszudrücken, abgebaut. Unterschiedliche Aktions- und Sozialformen ermöglichen zudem den Einsatz von kooperativen Lernformen, die in den Handreichungen für den Unterricht erläutert werden.

Die Grammatik in *Health Matters 3rd edition* ist auf das Wesentliche begrenzt. Grundlegende Strukturen werden in den Units im situativen Kontext vermittelt. Weitaus wichtiger sind jedoch die Erweiterung des berufsrelevanten Wortschatzes und das Erlernen feststehender Redewendungen, die als Rüstzeug für eine flüssige, effektive berufliche Kommunikation dienen.

Zur Vorbereitung auf die KMK-Prüfung für Niveau A2 und B1, werden in jeder Unit auf einer separaten Seite prüfungsrelevante Materialien und Aufgaben angeboten und so eine systematische Prüfungsvorbereitung ermöglicht.

Darüber hinaus finden Sie im Anhang eine komplette KMK-Musterprüfung (*mock exam*) für Niveau B1 sowie die Transkripte der Hörverständnistexte.

Sämtliche Audiomaterialien befinden sich in den Handreichungen für den Unterricht.

Abgerundet wird das Lehrwerk mit chronologischen und alphabetischen Wörterverzeichnissen sowie einer Grundwortschatzliste, die etwa 500 Wörter enthält, die für die Arbeit mit *Health Matters 3rd edition* als bekannt vorausgesetzt werden.

Der Verlag, der Autor und die Beraterin wünschen Ihnen viel Erfolg und Freude bei der Arbeit mit *Health Matters 3rd edition.*

Table of contents

Appendix

1 My workplace

1 Some typical activities for a medical assistant

A Match the duties below with these photos.

assist a doctor • keep patient records • look after patients • make telephone appointments • prepare surgical instruments and equipment • take blood samples

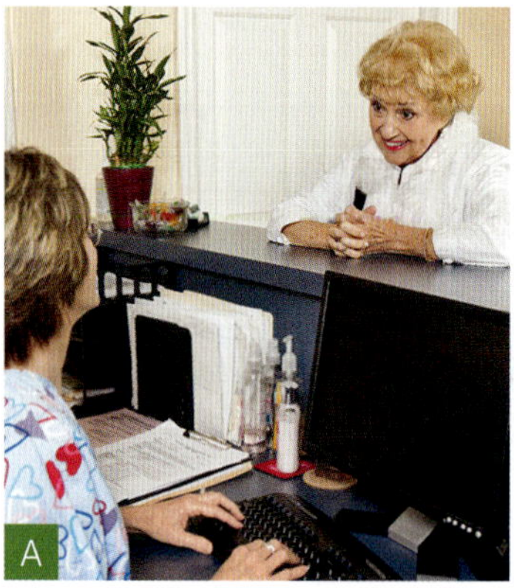
A

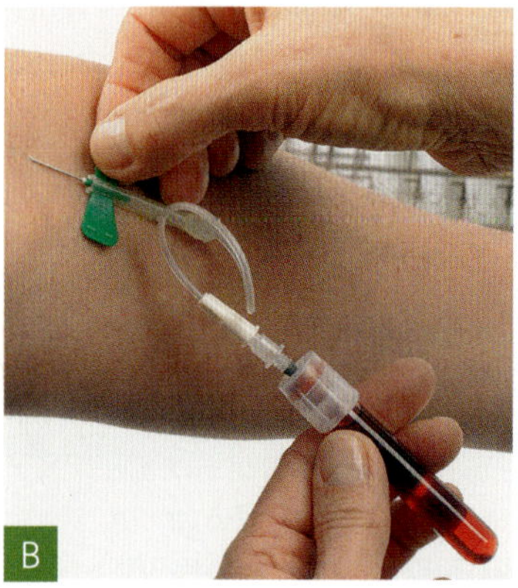
B

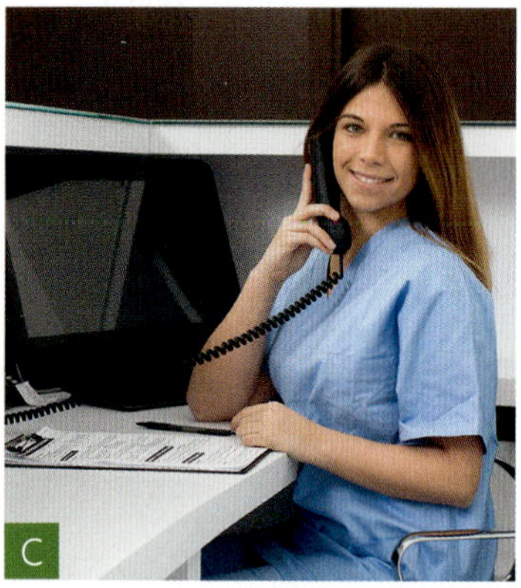
C

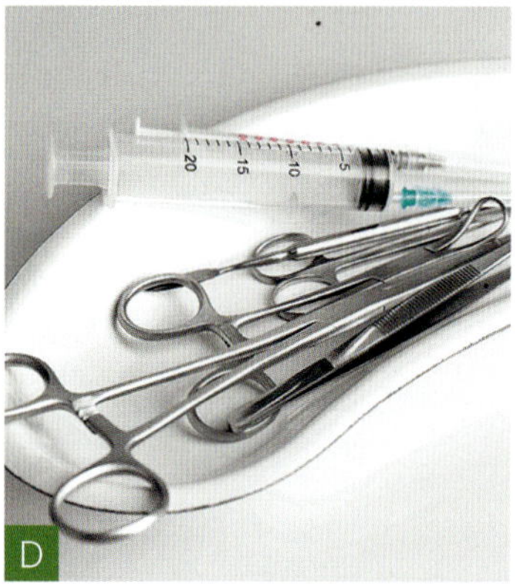

D

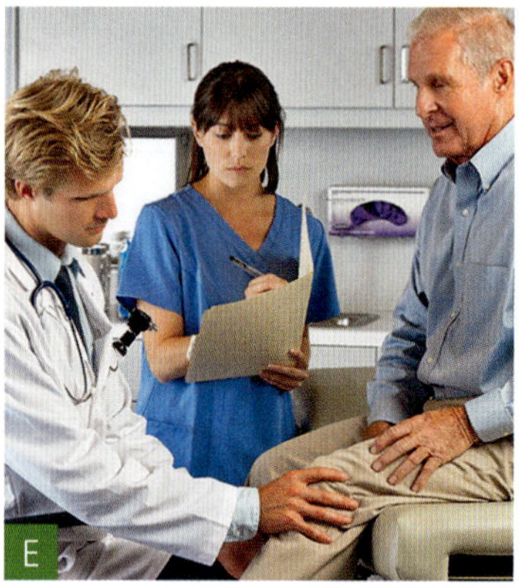
E

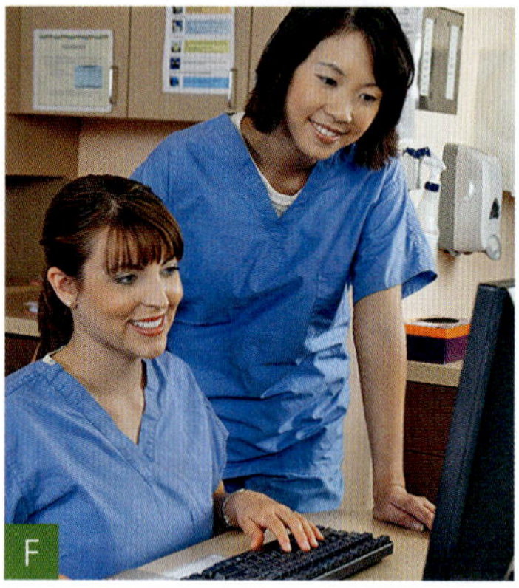
F

B Which of these duties do you do at work?

2 Describing duties

A The daily duties of a medical assistant can be put into the following groups.

Which do you like doing? Explain why.

- **a** Patient care
- **b** Organising the surgery and surgery hours
- **c** Assisting the doctor
- **d** Instrument care
- **e** Laboratory work
- **f** Office administration

> ! surgery (BE)
> doctor's office (AE)

B 02 Listen to some medical assistants talk about their work. Match the following statements and the daily duties.

1 One of the most important parts of the job is making sure the doctor has everything she needs when she's treating patients. So I make sure everything is OK and that the instruments are sterile and in the right place.

2 The front desk area is the first thing that patients see when they walk into the centre, so it has to look professional but also comfortable. So every day, before the first patients come, I make sure it's clean and tidy.

3 My favourite part of the job is working with people. When they come to the centre, they are often anxious or upset, so I try to be very friendly and calm and make them relax.

4 One part of my job I don't enjoy is doing all those tests. It's really boring analysing all the samples, and you have to be so careful you don't make a mistake.

5 I really like working with the doctor when he does minor operations. It's really exciting and I really enjoy watching him work. I help him and take notes. He's always so calm and relaxed.

6 I spend a lot of time doing paperwork such as preparing invoices and keeping patient records up to date. I also do the accounts and order supplies and things. Oh, and I'm also responsible for the surgery website and keep that up to date, too!

C Work with a partner. What other professional duties can you think of?

CULTURE

Health care

In the UK a doctor who works in a health centre and not in a hospital is called a GP (General Practitioner). You must be registered with a GP in order to receive healthcare. So when British people move house, they have to register with a new GP.

In the USA a General Practitioner is called a Primary Care Physician (PCP). People with general health insurance also have to register with a Primary Care Physician and go to that doctor first with any medical problem.

So you may find British and American patients ask to register with a doctor in Germany, too.

D Which verbs (1–8) go with the nouns (a–h)?

1	do	a	appointments
2	make	b	supplies
3	keep	c	patients
4	register with	d	patient records
5	prepare	e	paperwork
6	treat	f	a doctor
7	order	g	blood samples
8	take	h	instruments

E Here are some typical expressions that medical assistants need.

Which is the odd one out? Give a reason for your choice.

	a	b	c	d
1 do	paperwork	operations	instruments	tests
2 make	sure	appointments	a mistake	samples
3 keep	a website	records	up to date	calm
4 take	blood	records	samples	notes
5 prepare	invoices	paperwork	instruments	surgery
6 look after	patients	instruments	sterile	records

3 Describing your job

A Complete the sentences with the correct words from the list.

anxious · comfortable · sterile · tidy · friendly · calm · boring · up to date

1. I really don't like working in the lab. It's so ___.
2. I make sure all the instruments are ___ before they can be used.
3. I'm always very ___ with the patients and try to smile a lot.
4. Some patients get very ___ so I always explain everything to them.
5. It is important to have a ___ waiting room so that people feel relaxed when waiting for the doctor.
6. The doctor is very ___ and does everything very carefully.
7. I always ask patients to check their details so our records are ___.
8. Before I go home I make sure my desk is ___ for the next day.

B Work with a partner. Tell your partner about your job.

LANGUAGE

Describing your job
One of the most important parts of my job is …
Every day I …
I'm responsible for …
The favourite part of my job is …
The thing I find really interesting is …
One part of my job I don't enjoy is …
I really like …
I spend a lot of time …

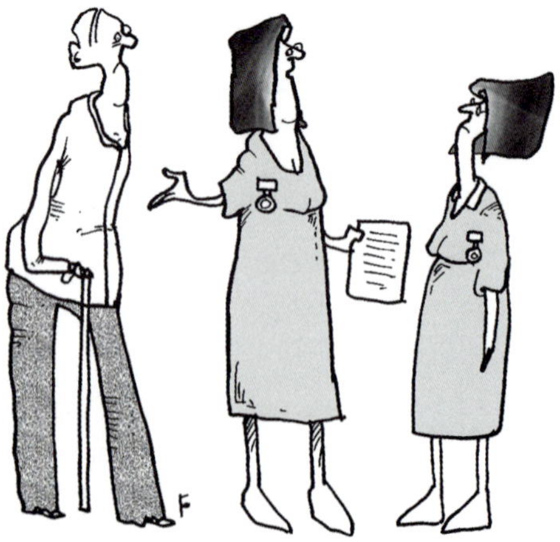

It's important to treat all our patients as INDIVIDUALS...this for example is individual number 78/gh5-fg34C.

Simple present (Die einfache Gegenwart)

1 I **make** appointments.
2 I **don't** (= **do not**) **take** X-rays.
3 The receptionist **greets** patients.
4 She **doesn't** (= **does not**) **like** lab work.
5 **Do** the patients **pay** in cash? – No, they **don't**.
6 **Does** the medical assistant **prepare** invoices? – Yes, she **does**.

- Das *simple present* wird für gleichbleibende Zustände, feststehende Tatsachen und regelmäßig sich wiederholende Handlungen verwendet.
- Bei *he/she/it* wird in der Regel *-(e)s* an die Grundform des Verbs angehängt. (3)
- Fragen und Verneinungen werden mit dem Hilfsverb *do* bzw. in der 3. Person Singular mit der Form *does* gebildet. (2, 4, 5, 6)
- In der Kurzantwort wird das Hilfsverb des Fragesatzes wiederholt. (5, 6)

4 Practice

With the information below, make complete sentences using the simple present.

1 the receptionist / register / patients
Example: *The receptionist registers patients.*
2 the nurse / collect / fees from private patients
3 good receptionists / work / well under pressure
4 medical assistants / need / excellent telephone skills
5 most patients / read / one of the magazines / the waiting room
6 the nurse / keep / medical supplies / this room
7 the receptionist / tidy / the waiting room / each morning
8 practices / always keep / old paper records
9 I / keep / website / up to date
10 the nurse / sometimes / do / paperwork / weekends

5 Practice

With the information below, make complete negative sentences or questions using the simple present.

1 the doctor / not make / appointments
Example: *The doctor does not (doesn't) make appointments.*
2 I / not take / X-rays
3 the medical assistants / not diagnose / general health problems
4 we / not make / paper records / any more
5 Dr Henderson / visit / her patients?
6 you / make / the coffee / in your surgery?
7 the practice / have / an electronic booking system?
8 you / finish / work / early on Friday?
9 a lot of patients / not like / injections
10 what / you / do / with / blood samples?

6 Giving directions

Joanna works at a health centre in London. A patient calls for directions to the centre.

A 03))) Listen to the recording and say what the letters A–F on the map refer to.

Archway · Ashbrook Road · Elthorne Road · Upper Holloway · Holloway Road · Fairbridge Road

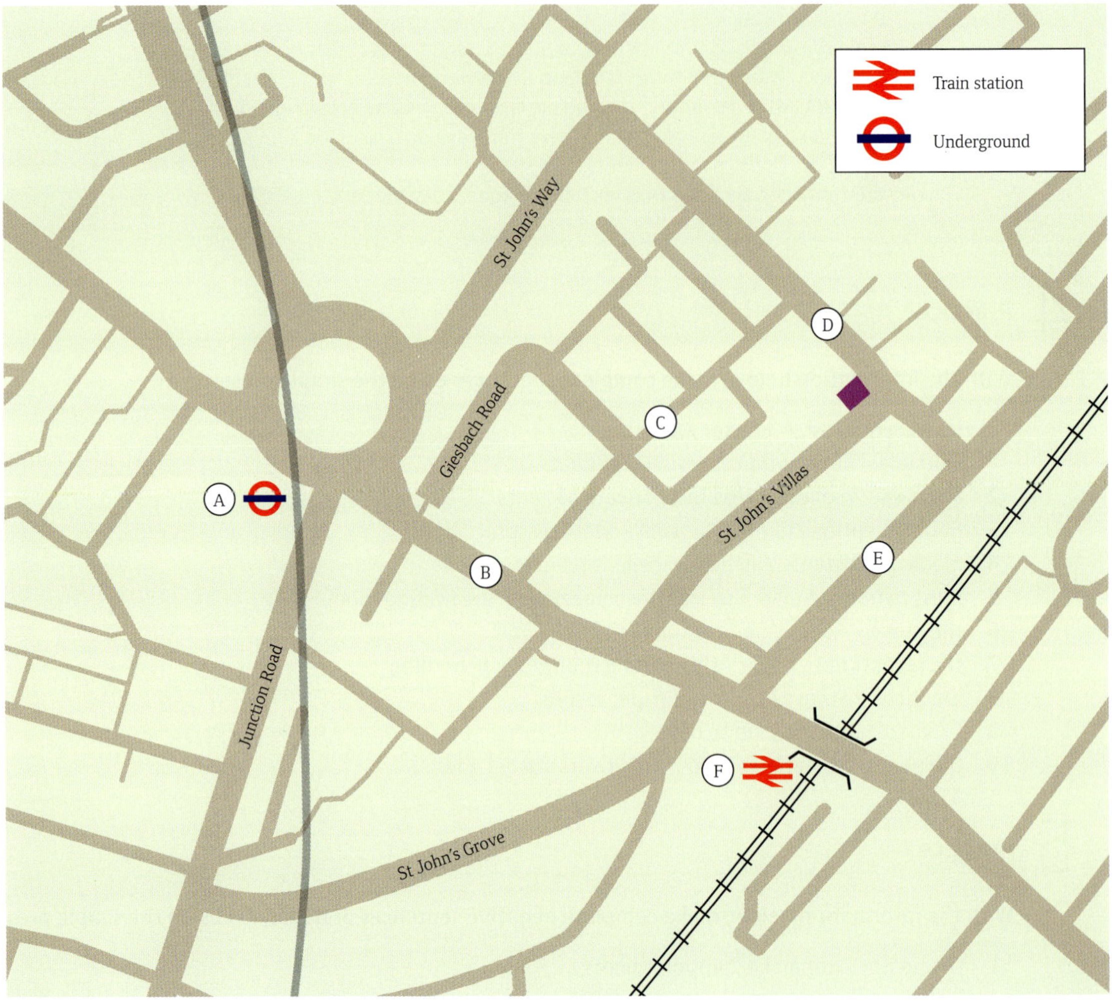

B Work with a partner. Draw a map for the practice where you work with street names and underground stations or bus stops. Give the map to your partner. Then tell your partner how to get to your practice. Your partner then marks it on your map.

LANGUAGE

Giving directions
Can you tell me how to get to ..., please?
Excuse me, please. Can you tell me where the ... is?
Take the train/underground/bus to ...
Go straight on and then turn left/right.
Take the (the first/second) left/right.
It's next to / between / opposite / on the corner of ...

7 Interaktion: A2

Situation: Sie sind vor Kurzem umgezogen und suchen einen Facharzt / eine Fachärztin in Ihrer Nähe. Sie machen sich im Internet kundig und sehen sich die Homepages einiger Arztpraxen an. Sie sehen Bilder von Medizinischen Fachangestellten.

→ Diskutieren Sie in der Fremdsprache mit einem Partner, ob deren Aussehen positive oder negative Auswirkungen auf Ihre Wahl der Praxis hat. Begründen Sie Ihre Meinung.

8 Leseverstehen: B1

Situation: Im Rahmen eines internationalen Austauschprogramms erwarten Sie in Ihrer Praxis in ca. zwei Wochen eine Praktikantin aus Manchester. Sie spricht nur wenig Deutsch. Um mit ihr besser kommunizieren zu können, beschäftigen Sie sich mit Texten aus dem Internet über „Medical Assistants“. Heute fanden Sie den unten stehenden Text. Über dessen Thema möchten Sie sich mit ihr austauschen.

→ Lesen Sie sich den Text genau durch und sammeln die im Text gegebenen Ratschläge in einer Positiv- und einer Negativliste. Anschließend verfassen Sie mit Hilfe Ihrer Mitschülerinnen bzw. Mitschüler eine Wandzeitung zu den „Dos and Don’ts of Appearance and Dress Codes in Medical Jobs“.

Appearance and Dress Codes in Medical Jobs

The reputation of a practice does not only depend on the doctors’ abilities, but also depends on the friendliness and helpfulness of its employees. But what about their appearance? What impression does a receptionist with greasy, unwashed hair make? How should make-up be used? What about the right clothing?

Most medical institutions have rules about “acceptable” clothes. Forget the image of a nurse in a white dress, shoes and hat. Most of today’s healthcare professionals wear “scrubs” – a general expression for any medical uniform consisting of loose, short-sleeved shirts paired with pants that have a drawstring. “Scrubs” got their name from being the clothing for a clean, or “scrubbed” environment. Years ago, medical workers wore white uniforms to symbolize cleanliness. After a while green uniforms became standard. Nowadays, you can find medical assistants wearing scrubs of different colors.

Medical assistants should wear comfortable footwear, such as athletic or walking shoes, suitable for spending long hours on their feet. Sandals, flip-flops and other open-toed shoes are unsuitable. These styles present a potential danger, for example, when fluids or heavy items are dropped. Socks are essential.

Do not wear hats or head coverings unless required for medical, cultural or religious reasons. Medical assistants should practise good personal hygiene and have a cultivated, professional appearance. Minimize or completely avoid using perfume. Maintain trimmed fingernails to reduce the risk of passing on infections. Make-up should be applied to look radiant, not provocative.

Employees should wear as little jewelry as possible to avoid potential injury. Many medical offices limit body piercing to the ears, with small earrings. In many clinics and medical practices medical assistants are often asked to cover their tattoos with long sleeves, make-up or bandages. If you are not sure about the appropriateness of your tattoo, you should speak to your supervisor or your employer.

9 Medical receptionist training in the UK

Your boss wants to know more about medical receptionist training in the United Kingdom.

A Read the text and note the important points about the qualifications and training. Then describe the situation in Germany and the UK.

Medical Reception Intermediate Diploma (AMSPAR*)

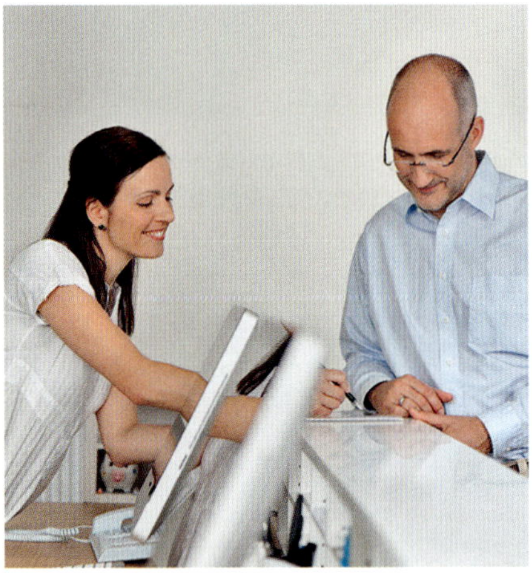

Are you caring and do you enjoy working with and for others? Do you enjoy working as part of a team? If the answers are yes, then you could be an ideal person to work in medical administration.

Medical receptionists play a very important role within a health care environment. They are part of the 'front line' staff and often the first person a patient or relative speaks to, either by telephone or in person. They are also involved in the electronic 'Choose and Book' scheme, where patients can make an appointment. The impression they make on people affects their opinion of the organization that they work for.

Medical receptionists can choose to work within general practice, hospitals, clinics or private practice. Studying for the AMSPAR Medical Reception Intermediate Diploma will give you the knowledge and skills required for this interesting and challenging role.

To achieve the Diploma you must:
- gain a pass in three written examinations (in June)
- gain a pass in nationally set assignments
- satisfy the work experience requirements and pass the work-based assignment

The programme is available for full or part-time study. The average length of the course is 12 months and is suitable for both school leavers and mature students.

* AMSPAR: The Association of Medical Secretaries, Practice Managers, Administrators and Receptionists

B Match the words (1–8) from the text with the definitions (a–h).

1 caring	a people who work for an organization
2 staff	b thinking about what other people need or want
3 relative	c what you think about something/someone
4 involved in	d piece of work given as part of a job
5 opinion	e member of your family
6 skill	f part of
7 required	g the ability to do something well
8 assignment	h needed

10 Medical office receptionist training in the USA

Now your boss wants to know about the situation in the USA.

A Read the website about medical office receptionist training in the USA and answer the questions below.

MOR

Medical Office Receptionist Certificate Programs

Certificate programs cover the very basic aspects needed to perform in the position of a medical receptionist. These are the key skills typically used in the field, including medical language, documentation and patient scheduling. Some certificate programs might require applicants to have certain levels of experience or education. Classes common to most medical office receptionist certificate programs cover these topics:

- Medical law and ethics
- Health care delivery
- Medical office accounting
- Business communications

Medical Office Receptionist Associate's Degree Programs

Associate's degree programs generally take two years to complete and include general education classes, along with the medical office coursework. Students who successfully complete the program will also be equipped with general anatomy knowledge, basic first aid and medical correspondence skills. In addition to classroom instruction, many associate's degree programs require students to complete on-site supervised internships at a medical office. Most associate's degree programs include the following:

- Basic clinical assisting methods
- Medical office emergency situations and procedures
- Clinical assisting in family practice settings
- Insurance processes and procedures
- Medical office patient records

1 What do you need before you start a medical office receptionist certificate program in the USA?
2 What coursework does a certificate program usually include?
3 Where does the training for the associate's degree program usually take place?
4 What are the differences between the two programs?
5 Which of the two programs would you like to do and why?

B Describe the differences in training and qualifications between Germany and the USA.

C As you have several English-speaking patients, your boss asks you to put some information on your health centre's website in English about how to become a medical assistant. He wants to employ an assistant from Britain or the USA.

Include the following:
- skills you need
- types of training
- qualifications

2 Making an appointment

1 Making telephone appointments

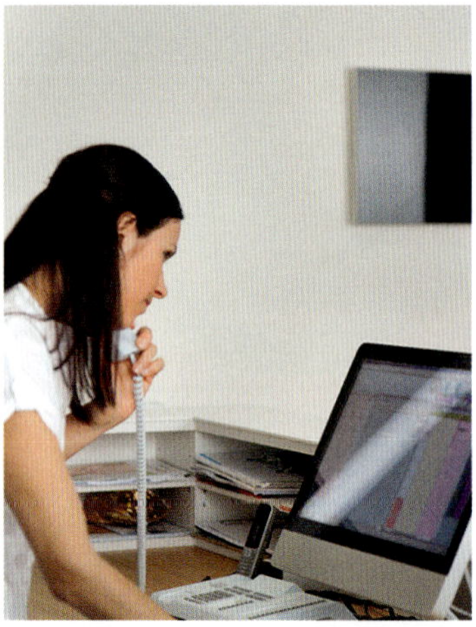

Kerstin Vogt works at a health centre in Passau. A British patient, Tony Collins, phones to make an appointment.

04 **First listen to the dialogue and do the exercise below. Then read and check your answers.**

Kerstin	Arztpraxis Stadtmitte. Guten Tag. Sie sprechen mit Frau Vogt.
Tony	Ah, hello. Can you speak English? Sorry, but my German isn't very good.
Kerstin	Yes, I can. Can I help you?
Tony	Oh good. Yes, I'd like to make an appointment, please.
Kerstin	No problem. Do you need an urgent appointment?
Tony	No, I don't think so. Tomorrow is OK.
Kerstin	OK, then let me have a look at what we have tomorrow. Could I have your name, please?
Tony	It's Collins. Mr Tony Collins.
Kerstin	OK. Would you like a morning or an afternoon appointment, Mr Collins?
Tony	Err, afternoon, please. Is late afternoon possible after work?
Kerstin	Let me see … We can fit you in at half four. Is that any good?
Tony	Yes, that's great. Thanks. Oh, err, sorry, can I just check that half four means half past four?
Kerstin	Yes, that's right, it's half past four tomorrow. Four thirty p.m. with Dr Müller. Have you got health insurance, Mr Collins?
Tony	Yes, I have an EHIC card*. I hope that's all right.
Kerstin	Yes, that's fine, no problem. See you tomorrow, Mr Collins.
Tony	Thank you. Goodbye.
Kerstin	You're welcome. Goodbye.

* The EHIC is the European Health Insurance Card which covers any necessary medical treatment due to an accident or illness within the European Economic Area. The card entitles the holder to state-provided medical treatment within the country they are visiting.

Are these statements true or false? Correct the false statements.

1. Tony can't speak any German.
2. His medical problem isn't very bad.
3. He can't do a morning appointment.
4. Kerstin makes an appointment for half past three.
5. Tony is registered with a German health insurance company.

CULTURE

Please, thank you* and *sorry

- British people use expressions of politeness such as *please* and *thank you* a lot.
- They also say *sorry* very often if they inconvenience someone.
- When you give someone something and they say thank you, the correct response is *You're welcome*, and not ~~*Please*~~.

LANGUAGE

Talking about appointments
Your appointment is for/at three forty-five.
We can fit you in at 8:15. a.m.
Is 7 o'clock in the evening OK?
Can you make half ten tomorrow morning?

- Die Zeitangabe *o'clock* wird nur bei einer vollen Stunde benutzt, z. B. *seven o'clock* = sieben Uhr.
- Auf Deutsch bedeuten *half past ten*, *half ten* und *ten thirty* alle halb elf.
- a.m. = vormittags, p.m. = nachmittags

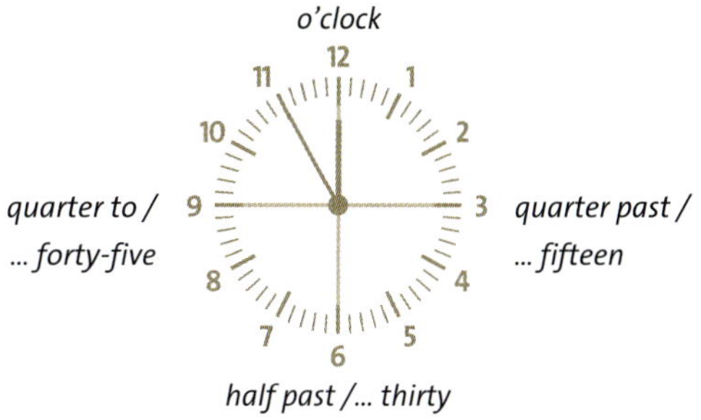

2 Telling the time

Match the times 1–10 with a–j.

1	twenty past ten	a	10:15
2	eleven o'clock	b	11:30
3	half past eleven	c	16:50
4	ten fifteen	d	10:20
5	eighteen fifteen	e	11:00
6	twenty to eleven	f	11:20
7	quarter to eleven	g	18:15
8	half past ten	h	10:30
9	eleven twenty	i	10:40
10	sixteen fifty	j	10:45

3 What time is it?

Kerstin has a friend, Sarah, who is a receptionist at the Epping Health Centre in the UK. She is making appointments with patients over the phone.

05 Listen and choose the correct appointment times.

1 10:30 / 11:30
2 4:50 / 4:15
3 12:10 / 11:50
4 8:45 / 9:15
5 8:30 / 9:30

4 Making appointments

Sarah makes four more appointments with patients.

06 Listen and write down the appointment times.

Patient	Appointment time

5 What's in the appointment book?

Work with a partner. Use the information and the phrases from exercises 2, 3 and 4 to make short dialogues.

Simple present forms of *be, have got*

1 **I'm** fine, you**'re** fine, but Tom **isn't**.
2 **Is** your appointment for today or tomorrow? – It**'s** for today.
3 **Are** you in pain? – Yes, I **am**./No, I**'m not**.
4 **I've got** my EHIC card, but I **haven't got** my prescription.
5 **Has** she **got** her health insurance card with her?
6 **Have** you **got** your prescription?

be
- Im Präsens hat das Verb drei Formen: *am, is, are*. (1, 2, 3)
- Die negativen Formen sind *'m not (am not), isn't, aren't*. (1, 3)
- Bei Fragen wird das Verb an den Satzanfang gestellt. (2, 3)

have got
- Im Präsens gibt es zwei Formen: *has got, have got* (oft zu *'ve* abgekürzt). (4)
- Die Negativformen sind *hasn't got, haven't got*. (4)
- Bei Fragen wird *has* oder *have* an den Satzanfang gestellt. (5, 6)

6 Practice

Complete the sentences with the correct form of the verbs. Write two more sentences.

1 The appointment ___ (be) for 8:45 on Thursday.
2 We ___ (not / be) very busy today.
3 ___ (be) Mr Bell in the waiting room?
4 I ___ (be) sorry, but you ___ (be) too late for your appointment.
5 I'm sorry but I ___ (not / have got) an appointment.
6 ___ (she/have got) her insurance card with her?
7 ___ (you/have got) your prescription?
8 Dr Thomas ___ (not/have got) the results of your blood test yet.
9 ___
10 ___

7 Spelling names

Kerstin's school friend, Lara, works at a health centre in Frankfurt. Many foreign patients come to the centre and Lara has to make sure she spells their names correctly.

07 **Listen to the dialogues and choose the correct spelling.**

1	**a** Gawlinski	**b** Gelinski	**c** Gawlinka
2	**a** Tunchi	**b** Tuncay	**c** Toonshy
3	**a** Kusnetzof	**b** Kasnestof	**c** Kuznetsov
4	**a** Yildirim	**b** Yedilim	**c** Yidrilm
5	**a** Wizocksi	**b** Wysocki	**c** Wiysoke
6	**a** Leigh	**b** Leegh	**c** Liegh

Work with a partner. Spell your names to each other.

8 Telephone etiquette

The way a medical assistant answers the phone and deals with callers is a very important part of the image of a surgery.

A **Look at the procedure below and match the reasons with the steps.**

- **a** This allows you to call the patient back in case you get disconnected.
- **b** This treats patients with courtesy – especially when asking them to wait.
- **c** So the medical assistant knows who the patient is.
- **d** This shows you are happy to help the caller and not trying to end the call quickly.
- **e** So the medical assistant knows if it is an emergency.
- **f** Answering promptly gives a professional image.
- **g** This confirms that the caller has the correct number and knows who they are speaking to.
- **h** The caller can't see it but will hear it in your voice.

STEPS	REASONS
Step 1: Answer the phone.	
1 Smile before you answer.	
2 Answer by the third ring.	
3 Speak clearly, identify yourself and the centre.	
4 Identify the name of the caller.	
5 Provide the service or information the caller needs.	Medical assistants deal with many types of call and save the doctor a lot of time.
Step 2: If necessary, put a caller on hold.	
6 Ask permission to put a caller on hold.	
Step 3: If necessary, take a message.	
7 Note the time, the date and who the message is for.	So the message goes to the right person and they know when the call was made.
8 Note the name of the caller and a contact number.	
9 Note the urgency of the message.	
Step 4: Close the call.	
10 Offer further assistance.	
11 Thank the caller by name.	Saying 'Thank you for calling, Mrs Jones. Good-bye.' shows courtesy and respect.

B **Work with a partner. Practise making calls using the etiquette in the table.**

9 Dealing with a new patient

Candy Donnelly is Australian but lives in Passau. She phones Dr Müller's surgery to make a first appointment.

Look at the box below. What does Kerstin say?

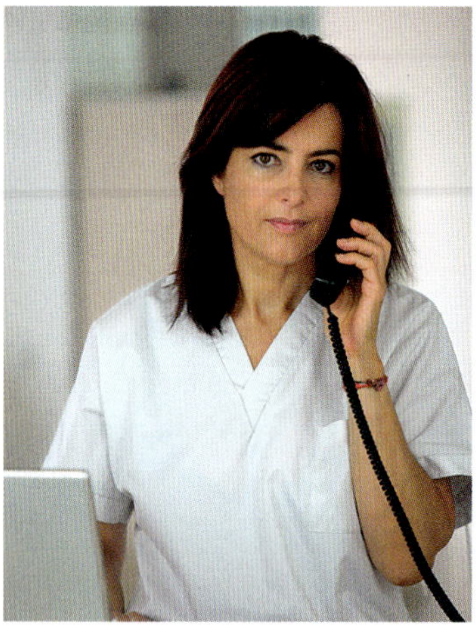

Kerstin	Arztpraxis Stadtmitte. Guten Tag. Sie sprechen mit Frau Vogt.
Candy	Oh hello, can you speak English?
Kerstin	___ 1
Candy	Oh good. Can I make an appointment, please?
Kerstin	___ 2
Candy	Yes, it is.
Kerstin	___ 3
Candy	It's Candy Donnelly. That's D-O-double N-E-double L-Y.
Kerstin	___ 4
Candy	It's 24th February 1996.
Kerstin	___ 5
Candy	It's Theresienstraße 32.
Kerstin	___ 6
Candy	It's 94032 Passau.
Kerstin	___ 7
Candy	It's 8955236.
Kerstin	___ 8
Candy	Yes, I have.
Kerstin	___ 9
Candy	Yes, Friday morning, please. Can I have an early appointment?
Kerstin	___ 10
Candy	Yes, that's a good time. Thanks.
Kerstin	___ 11
Candy	That's no problem. I can come a bit early.
Kerstin	Good. Thank you. So, see you on Friday, Ms Donnelly. Goodbye.

CULTURE

Use of first names

In general, people in the UK and USA address each other with first names, even in formal work situations when speaking to colleagues.
But in customer service situations it is normally polite to use titles such as Mr, Mrs or Ms followed by the surname when speaking to a customer or patient.

Kerstin

a Yes, I can. Can I help you?
b And the postcode, please?
c Thank you. And your address, please?
d That's great. Can you bring it with you, please? Now we need to make a first appointment. Is there any day or time you would like?
e 94032. Thank you. And your telephone number?
f Is this your first appointment with our practice?
g Good. So that's Friday, 18 June at twenty-five to nine. Can you come ten minutes early, please, as you need to complete a medical history form?
h Right, early. Let's have a look. Is 8:35 OK?
i Then I need to take some details first. So, can I have your full name, please?
j That's 8955236. And have you got a health insurance card?
k And your date of birth, please, Ms Donnelly?

10 A record file

Kerstin keys in Candy Donnelly's details. This is her patient file.

Copy it into your exercise book. Then read the dialogue again and write down the missing information.

Familienname:				Vorname:			
Geburtsdatum:							
Straße:		Hausnummer:		PLZ:		Stadt:	
Telefonnummer:							
Datum des Termins:		Tag:		Zeit:			
Kassenpatient:		Privatpatient:					
Krankenkasse/Versicherung:							

11 A new patient

A new patient walks into your practice. It's his/her first appointment.

Work with a partner and role-play a dialogue.

Medical assistant

Begrüßen Sie die neue Patientin/den neuen Patienten und fragen Sie, ob Sie helfen können.

Patient

Fragen Sie die/den MFA*, ob sie/er Englisch kann.

Medical assistant

Sagen Sie, dass Sie es können und fragen, ob sie/er einen Termin hat.

Patient

Sagen Sie Nein, und dass Sie das erste Mal zu diesem Arzt/dieser Ärztin gehen.

Medical assistant

Fragen Sie nach den nötigen persönlichen Daten. Überprüfen Sie die Schreibweisen.

Patient

Geben Sie Ihre persönlichen Daten an.

Medical assistant

Fragen Sie, wann die Patientin/der Patient gerne einen Termin hätte.

Patient

Machen Sie Ihren ersten Termin aus.

Medical assistant

Bestätigen Sie den Termin und verabschieden Sie sich.

Patient

Bedanken Sie sich bei der/dem MFA und verabschieden Sie sich.

* MFA = Medizinische/r Fachangestellte/r

12 08 Hörverstehen: A2

Situation: Sie sind Auszubildende/r als medizinische/r Fachangestellte/r in der Praxis Dr. Rose. Nach einem Feiertag an einem Dienstag hören Sie als Erstes den Anrufbeantworter ab. Es ist eine Mitteilung in englischer Sprache dabei, diese wird Ihnen drei Mal vorgespielt.
→ **Notieren Sie stichwortartig die Angaben des Anrufs auf einem Extrablatt.**

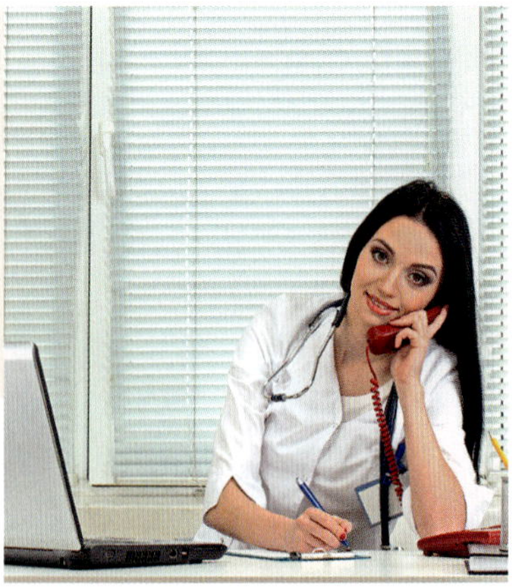

- Anrufer
- Grund für den Anruf
- Wünsche
- Rückmeldunq
- Sonstiges

13 09 Hörverstehen: B1

Situation: Sie sind Auszubildende/r als medizinische/r Fachangestellte/r in der Praxis Dr. Rose. Nach einem Feiertag an einem Dienstag hören Sie als Erstes den Anrufbeantworter ab. Es sind zwei Mitteilungen in englischer Sprache dabei. Diese werden Ihnen jeweils zwei Mal vorgespielt.
→ **Notieren Sie stichwortartig die Angaben der beiden Anrufe auf einem Extrablatt.**

	Anrufer 1	Anrufer 2
Name		
Grund für den Anruf		
Wünsche		
Rückmeldung		
Sonstiges		

14 Making appointments

A Look at the following information about how to see a GP in the UK and answer the questions below.

GP appointments and bookings

Visits to the surgery are free, but you'll usually need to make an appointment. Before you make an appointment to see your GP, consider the alternatives. Your local pharmacist may be able to give you the help you need, so you won't have to spend time waiting for an appointment. You can still phone the GP practice outside normal surgery hours, but you will usually be directed to an out-of-hours service. Alternatively, you can call NHS 111 if you urgently need medical help or advice but only if it's not a life-threatening situation.
Most GP practices have their own booking routines. Your surgery should be able to offer you an appointment to see a GP or other healthcare professional quickly, if necessary.

Home | Information ▾ | Practice Staff ▾ | Other Services ▾ | Health Advice ▾

Welcome to Linton Health Centre

To make an appointment with a doctor or nurse please telephone our appointments line on 01234 98765. You can also register at reception to use our online patient services. This will enable you to book/cancel appointments with a doctor and order repeat prescriptions online.

Extended Hours Surgeries

We offer three extended hours surgeries each week: Late evening surgeries (until 8 p.m.), early morning surgeries (from 6:30 a.m.), and an occasional Saturday morning surgery (8:30 a.m.–10:00 a.m.).
All extended hours surgeries are for pre-booked appointments only. There is no duty doctor and no emergency services during these sessions. The out-of-hours service provides an emergency service outside our normal working hours.

1 What alternatives are there to seeing a GP?
2 Name the three different ways of making an appointment.
3 What can you do if you need an appointment outside of surgery hours?
4 The health centre offers various online services – what are they?
5 What extra services does the health centre offer?

B Your practice is receiving more and more foreign patients. So your boss asks you to put some information on your website in English.

Include the following:
- surgery hours
- how to make an appointment
- any extra services

3 At reception

1 Paying for services

As part of your training you are asked to find out about how people pay for healthcare in the USA and UK so that you are in a position to explain in English how the system works in Germany to any foreign patient.

Read the two websites and then do the exercise at the top of page 23.

Paying for healthcare in the USA

In the USA there is public and private insurance coverage. About 62% of people in the USA have private medical insurance.
Doctors in the USA are called physicians and a general family doctor is called a Primary Care Physician. As the name suggests, this doctor will take care of your basic needs. If you need specialist treatment, the physician will refer you to a specialist. However, if you have private insurance, you can go straight to a specialist.
Whether you see a primary care physician or a specialist, you have to pay part of the cost, and this will be between $10–$50. The doctor will send the bill directly to the insurance company but will ask you to pay your share by credit card, check or in cash.
If you are tourist in the USA, it is different. In this case you pay the doctor in full (cash or credit card) and then claim back from your German insurance when you get back home.

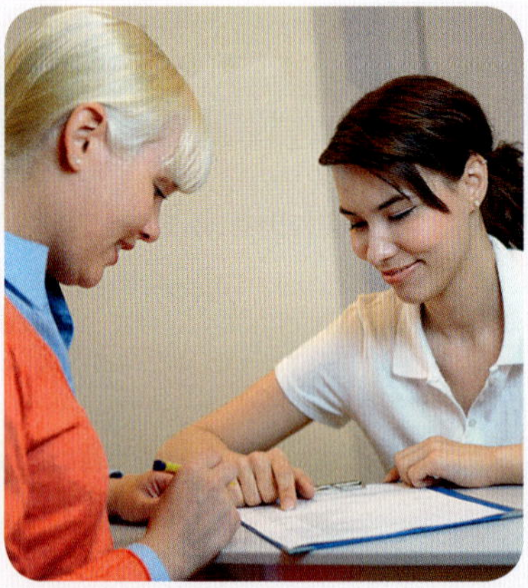

Paying for healthcare in the UK

In the UK taxpayers pay for the National Health Service (NHS), which provides all public healthcare in the UK including hospitals and general doctor services. This means that a visit to your family doctor is free of charge. Before seeing a doctor, you must register with the surgery and get an NHS Medical Card with an NHS Number. If you need some specialist healthcare, your GP will refer you to a hospital specialist. The current prescription charge is £8.40 (about €10) per item, which you pay directly to the pharmacy.

You can also get private health treatment for any medical condition in the UK, but it is quite expensive. Only about 10% of people in Britain have private health insurance.

As a tourist, you can go to a local health centre and be treated there. You do not have to pay: the NHS bears these costs.

Say whether the following statements are true for the UK, USA or both.

1 Some people have private health insurance.
2 You don't have to pay for a doctor's appointment.
3 You can pay the doctor directly in cash.
4 You have to register with a doctor.
5 You need a referral to see a specialist.
6 Tourists pay the doctor.

2 Healthcare in Germany

An American friend of yours is a doctor and visiting Germany on holiday.

A In pairs, make a dialogue using the information in the websites and the words below to explain to her how people pay for healthcare in Germany.

state insurance company · private insurance · charge · register · referral · specialist · treatment

B Now present your dialogue to the class.

3 Dealing with walk-ins

Kerstin is a medical assistant at a health centre in Passau. The following foreigners walk into the health centre and ask to see a doctor.

A 10 Listen and match the dialogues with the photographs.

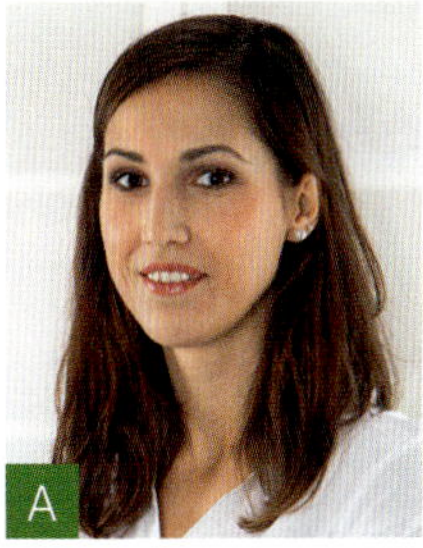
A

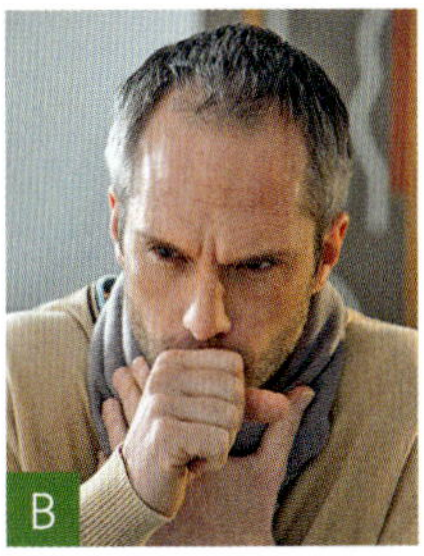
B

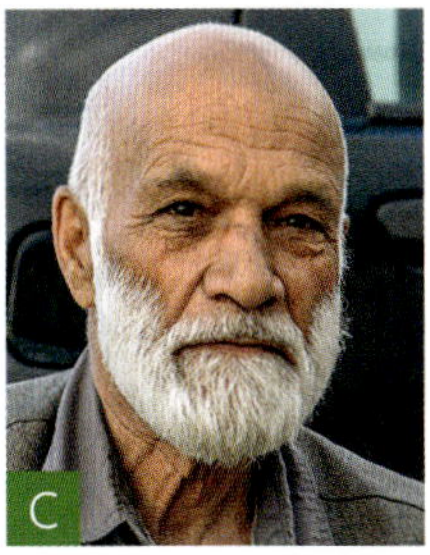
C

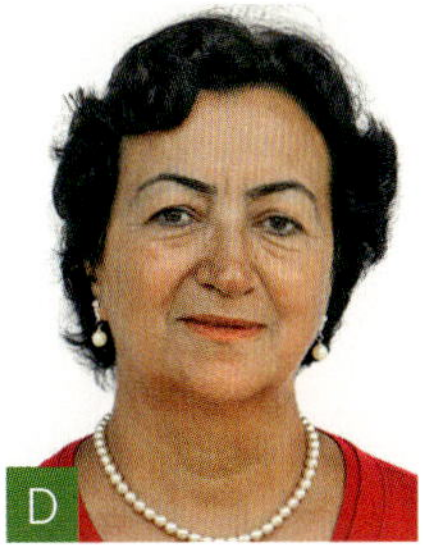
D

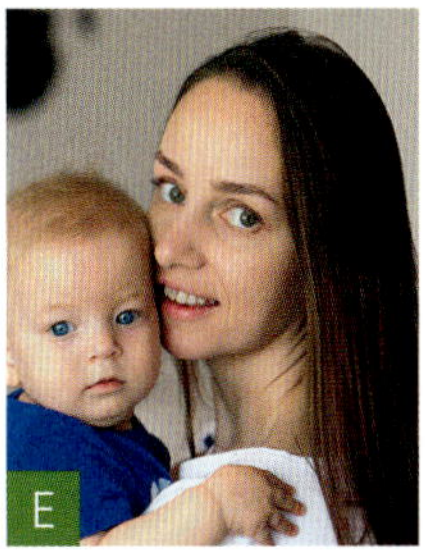
E

B Work with a partner. Copy the table into your exercise book. Listen again and make a note of what the problem is and how/when it happened. What action do you think Kerstin took in each case?

Case	Problem	How/When it happened	Action
Adnan Hussain			
Zeynap Yilmaz's mother			
Aleksandra Bartolski			
Gianna Bianchi			
Paul Clark			

C 11 Listen to what action Kerstin took. Look at your table again – were you right?

4 Working with words

In your exercise book, complete the sentences with the correct word.

sick · swollen · chest · fever · sore · pain

1 My finger was very ___, I couldn't get my wedding ring off.
2 I felt ___ and had a temperature.
3 She had a ___ in her stomach.
4 His ___ hurt and he couldn't breathe properly.
5 I spilled hot coffee on my arm and it's still a bit ___.
6 She has got a high temperature and a ___.

Simple past (Die einfache Vergangenheit)

1 It **happened** about an hour ago.
2 It **started** this morning.
3 He **breathed** in deeply when the doctor **listened** to his chest.
4 I **didn't** (= **did not**) **put** anything on it.
5 When **did** it **happen**?

- Das *simple past* wird für Handlungen gebraucht, die in der Vergangenheit völlig abgeschlossen wurden (oft mit Signalworten wie *last week*, *yesterday*, *ago* usw.). (1)
- Bei regelmäßigen Verben bildet man das *simple past*, indem man *-ed* oder *-d* an die Grundform anfügt. (1, 2, 3)
- Die Frageform wird mit *did* + Grundform (5), die Verneinung mit *didn't* + Grundform (4) gebildet.
- Eine Liste der unregelmäßigen Verben befindet sich auf Seite 143.

5 Practice

In your exercise book, complete the sentences with the correct form of the simple past.

1 The doctor ___ (tell) me to come back next week.
2 I ___ (make) an appointment for you on Thursday at 9 a.m. with Dr Marsh.
3 The patient ___ (wait) for an hour yesterday to see the doctor.
4 I ___ (receive) a letter from my GP last week.
5 The doctor ___ (refer) the patient to the local hospital.
6 She ___ (register) with her local health centre when she ___ (move) to her new house here.

6 Practice

Now complete these sentences with the correct negative or question form of the simple past.

1 She ___ (not / see) the doctor last week although her foot was very sore.
2 ___ (you / have) a blood test when you saw the doctor yesterday?
3 I ___ (not / get) an appointment last Friday because the surgery was so full.
4 ___ (the antibiotics / stop) the infection quickly?
5 ___ (you / take) your medicine when you got up this morning?
6 My GP ___ (not / know) what was wrong with me.

7 Giving directions

Kerstin's friend, Sarah, works in Epping Health Centre in Britain. Here is a floor plan of where she works.

A 12 Listen to the recording and match the rooms to the numbers. The patients are in the waiting room but walk into Reception and speak to Sarah and/or her colleague there.

Number … is/are the … treatment room 2/3 • patients' toilets • laboratory • X-ray room • office

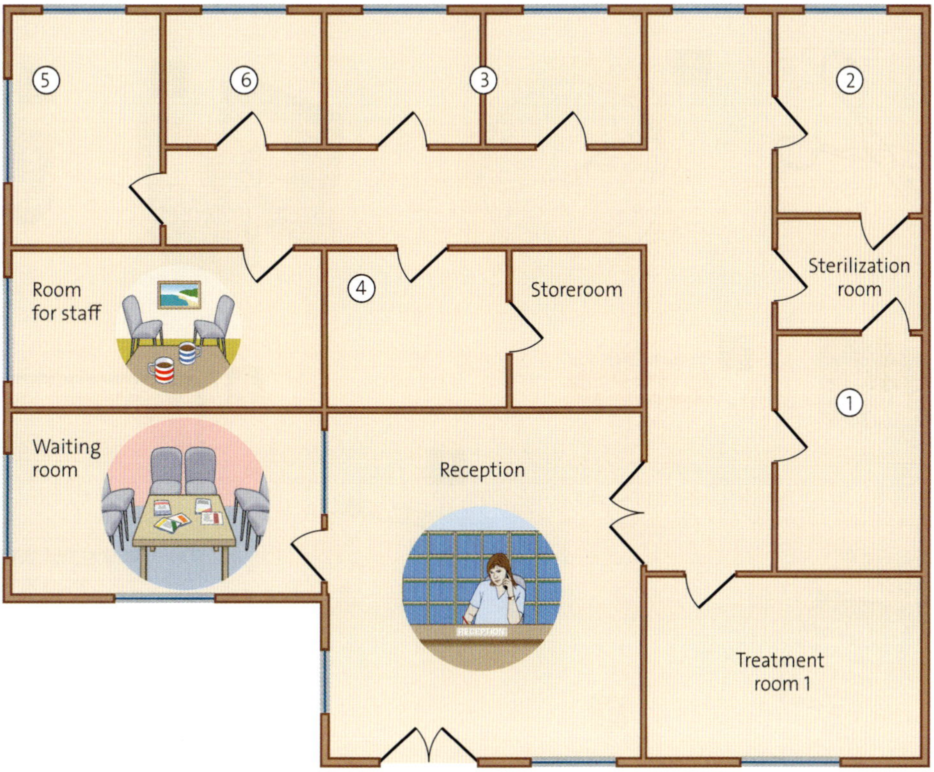

B Draw a floor plan of the practice where you work and label reception and one other room. Next to the plan, write the names of the other rooms in the practice.

C Work with a partner. Give the plan to your partner. Then help each other label the floor plans by asking for and giving directions. Always start at reception.

LANGUAGE

Giving directions in the practice

Go straight on and then turn left/right.
Go down/along the corridor.
Go up/down the stairs.
Go through the door(s) and …
It's just here in front of you.
It's (the first/second) door/room on the left/right.
It's next to/between/opposite the …

Where's the waiting room, please?

Excuse me, please. Can you tell me where the ___ is?

Excuse me, where is/are the ___ ?

8 Reception and office equipment

Sarah's sister, Emily, also works at a UK health centre. She is a receptionist there. One of her duties is to manage equipment supplies at the centre.

Match the words to the illustrations below.

electronic appointment book · appointment cards · calendar · card reader port · clock · calculator · keyboard · label printer · scissors · stapler · printer cartridges · copier paper

1
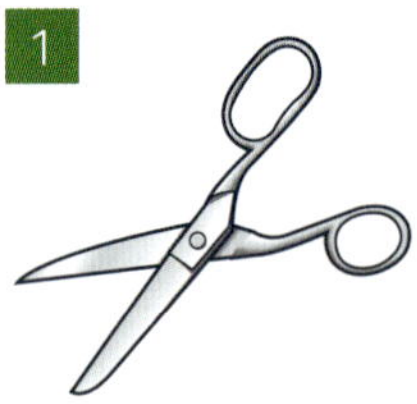

2
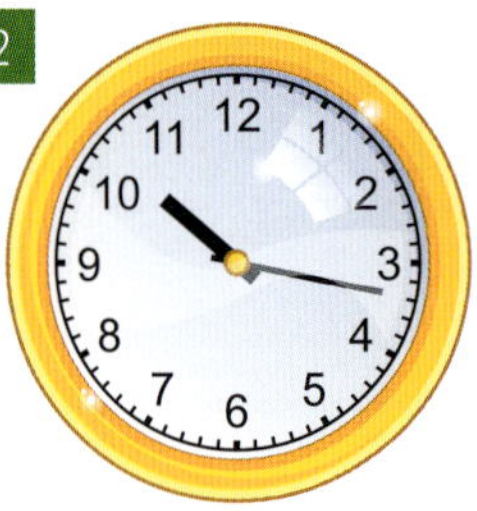

3
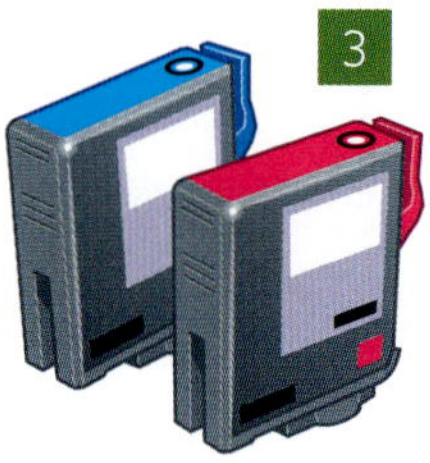

4
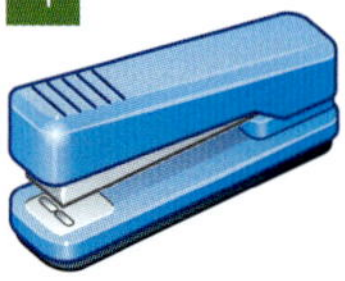

5
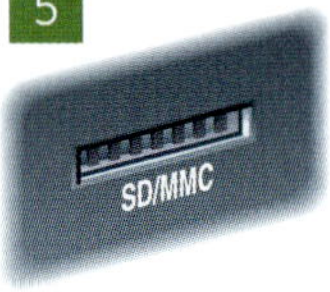

6
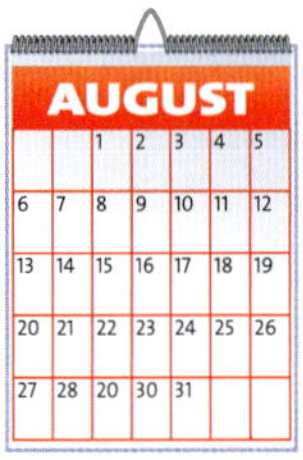

7
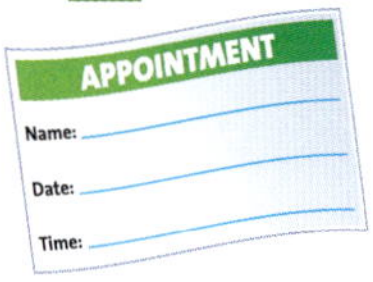

8
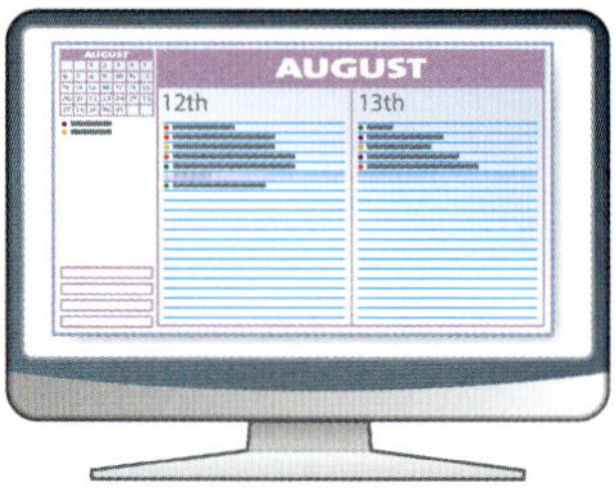

9
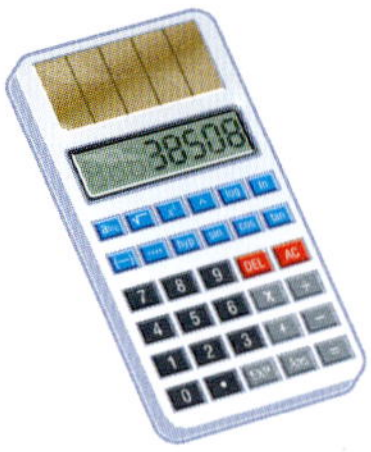

10
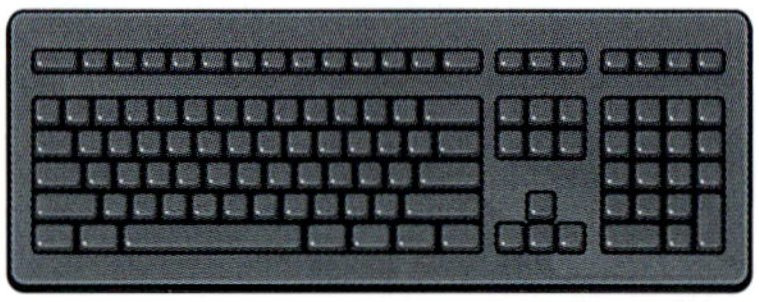

11
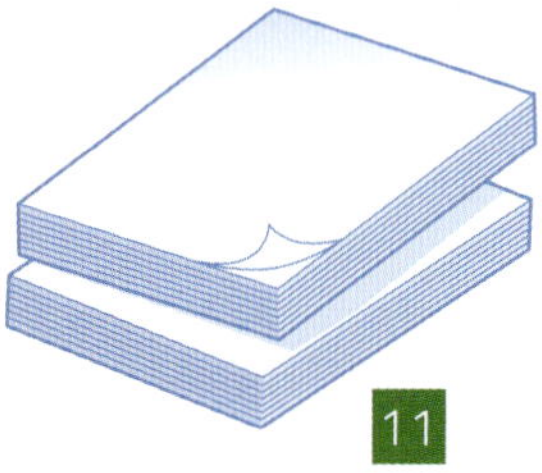

12
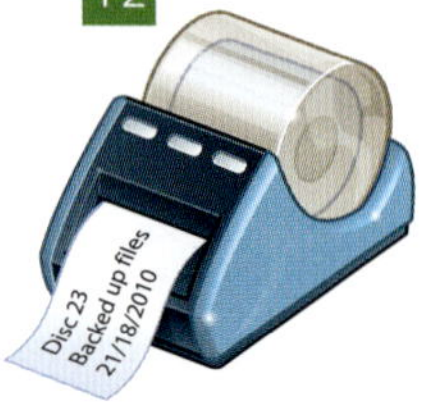

9 Working with words

Work with a partner. Use the words in the list to describe what you use the things from exercise 8 for.

write down appointment times · make appointments · check the date · print documents/labels · read medical insurance cards · cut things · key information into the system · attach pieces of paper together · do sums · check the time · make copies of documents · make printouts of documents

I use an electronic appointment book to ___.

We use ___ to ___.

We don't use a ___ to ___.

10 Ordering office equipment

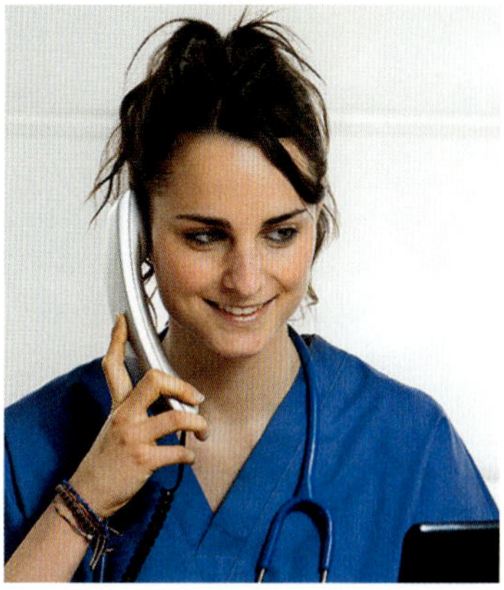

Today Emily is ordering some equipment for the health centre.

A 13))) Listen to the dialogue and then complete the conversation below.

John Good morning, Saxon Office Supplies. Can I help you?
Emily Yes, I'd like to make ___[1] order, please.
John OK, great. Do you have ___[2] customer reference number?
Emily Yes, it's 235432.
John And could I have the first line of your address, please?
Emily It's the Lea Valley Health Centre.
John And could I have your name, please?
Emily It's Emily Watson.
John OK Emily, my name's John. What would you like to order?
Emily I'd like ___[3] Post-It notes, please. The large ones. Do you have ___[4] packs with different colours?
John So that's the 76 x 127 size. They're in packs of 12. Ah, we don't have ___[5] of the coloured packs at the moment, I'm afraid. Only the yellow ones. Is that OK?
Emily That's fine. Can I have three packs, please?
John Of course. That's three packs at £18.99 each.
Emily I need ___[6] staples, too. The 26/6 ones.
John OK, they come in boxes of 5000 and cost £2.50 each. How many would you like?
Emily Five boxes, please. And I need ___[7] pens, too. Do you have ___[8] of those ballpoint Supergrip pens? Blue ones, please.
John We only have two boxes of the blue ones left, I'm afraid. Would you like ___[9] of the black ones? They're both £4.70 for a box of five.
Emily No, it's OK. Just the two blue ones, thanks.
John OK, anything else?
Emily Yes, one last thing. I need ___[10] HP364 printer cartridges. Do you have ___[11] of the XL size?
John One moment, 364 ___ we do, yes. Which colours do you need?
Emily Do you have ___[12] pack with all four colours?
John We do, in fact they're on special offer this week – £45.50 for a pack of four.
Emily Oh, that's good. Then, two packs please, and that's everything.
John Great, OK, so all together that comes to, let me see, …

B 13))) Look at Emily's list and listen to her order again. Then correct the list to show what she actually ordered and work out the total price.

a/an; some/any

1 Do you have **a** customer reference number, please?
2 I need **some** staples.
3 Do you have **any** of the XL size?
4 We don't have **any** of the coloured ones.

- Man verwendet *a/an*, wenn man sich auf einzelne Dinge, Personen usw. bezieht. (1)
- *Some* und *any* können sowohl bei zählbaren als auch bei nicht zählbaren Begriffen stehen. In Aussagesätzen wird *some* verwendet. (2)
- In Fragen (3) und verneinten Sätzen (4) wird *any* gebraucht.

- *Post-It notes (coloured, 3 packs)*
- *Staples (26/6, 5 boxes)*
- *Pens (ballpoint Supergrips, blue, 4 packs)*
- *Printer cartridges (HP364XL all 4 colours, one pack)*

11 Produktion

Situation: Die Praxis, in der Sie beschäftigt sind, wird in einem Monat für eine Woche wegen Renovierungs- und Wartungsarbeiten geschlossen. Da Sie viele Patienten haben, mit denen Sie auf Englisch kommunizieren, fertigen Sie für diese ein Hinweisschild an. Dieser Text soll auch auf der Internetseite der Praxis Verwendung finden.

→ **Schreiben Sie den englischen Text für Ihre Patienten. Er enthält folgende zusätzliche Angaben:**

- **Schließung vom 16.3. – 20.3.**
- **Vertretung: Dr. Walter**
- **Beschreibung des Wegs zu dessen Praxis**
- **die gleichen Öffnungszeiten**
- **Bitte um Verständnis**
- **Rezeptwünsche bitte rechtzeitig**

Benutzen Sie diesen Stadtplan für Ihre Wegbeschreibung.

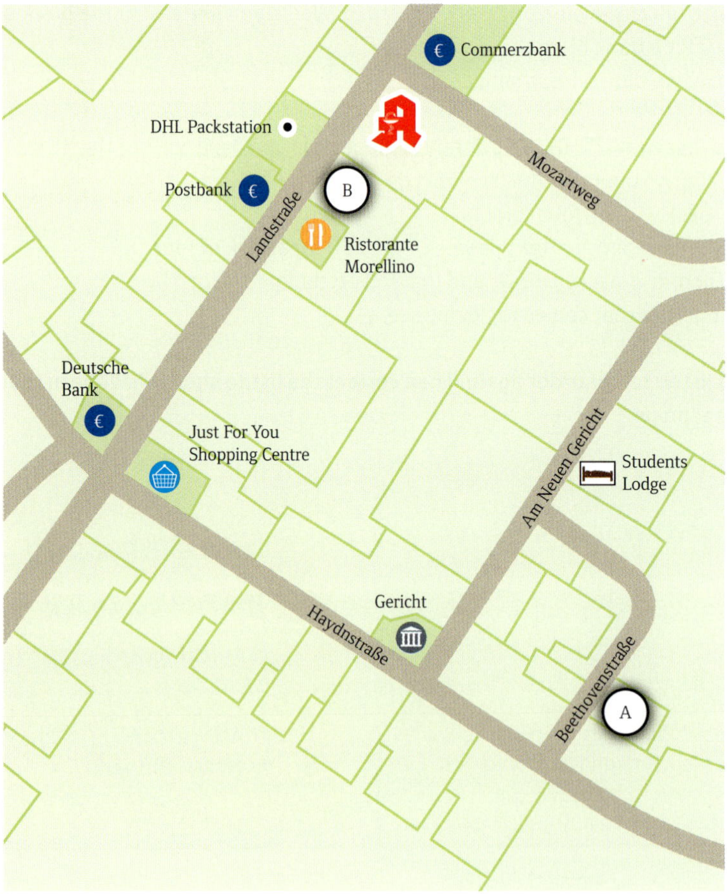

A = Ihre Praxis
B = Praxis von Dr. Walter

EM Extra Material

12 Basic personal information

You have a foreign visitor in your surgery. You need the following information:

Vorname · Familienname · Adresse in Deutschland · Geburtsdatum · Telefonnummer · Handynummer · Name der Versicherung · Krankheiten

How would you ask for this information in English?

13 Medical history

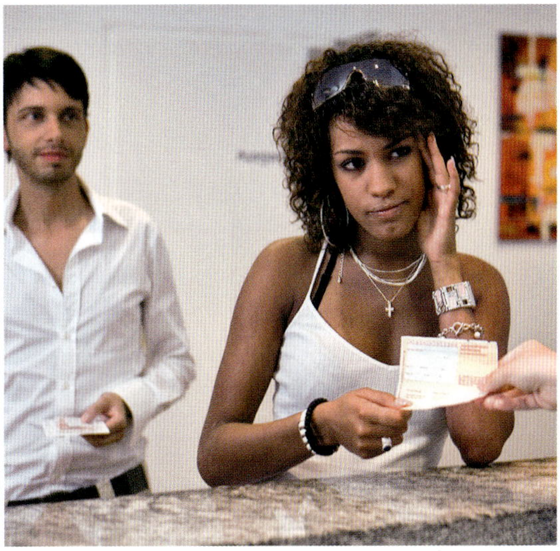

Your practice is getting more and more foreign patients. Your boss asks you to translate the practice medical history form into English.

14)) Listen to a medical assistant ask the questions in English and then use a dictionary and the words from the list below to help you write the questions in English.

medical treatment · allergic reaction · drugs · injections · tablets · medicine · pregnant · HIV positive · health problems · hepatitis B · anxious

1 Sind Sie zurzeit in ärztlicher Behandlung?
2 Hatten Sie jemals nach Einnahme von Medikamenten oder nach Spritzen oder Betäubungsmitteln eine allergische Reaktion?
3 Nehmen Sie zurzeit Medikamente? Wenn ja, welche?
4 Sind Sie schwanger?
5 Sind Sie HIV-positiv?
6 Wann war Ihr letzter Besuch in einer Arztpraxis?
7 Haben Sie im Moment irgendwelche gesundheitliche Probleme?
8 Haben Sie Hepatitis B?
9 Werden Sie während einer ärztlichen Behandlung ängstlich oder nervös?

LANGUAGE

Can you tell me …?
Have you ever …?
At the moment, are you …?
When was the last time you …?
Do you have …?
Are you (Do you get) nervous …?

4 Describing symptoms

1 Which type of doctor?

Katja works at a health centre that has several different kinds of doctors.

These six patients are in the waiting room. Look at the words below and decide who Katja sends the patients to.

general practitioner (GP) · gynaecologist · nurse · paediatrician · physiotherapist · radiologist

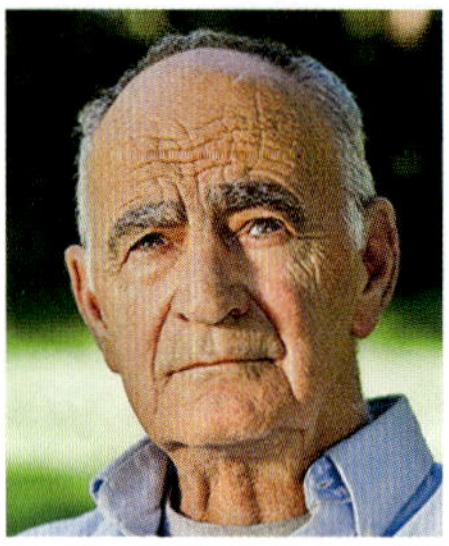

Harry Taylor
Eight weeks ago I fell down some stairs and broke my leg. It was a very bad break, so now I have to learn to walk again without crutches.
I come here almost every day.

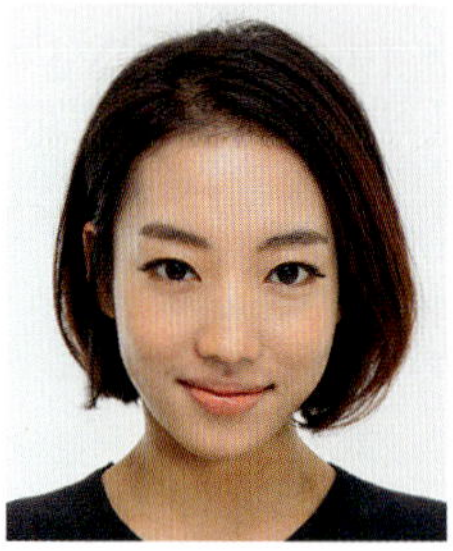

Cindy Wong
I keep getting migraines, so I went to my GP but she didn't know what was wrong. So, she sent me here to get some scans of my head.

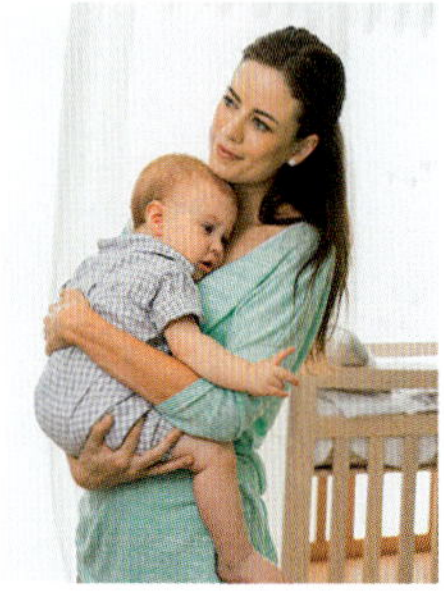

Birgül and Erkan Yildiz
I'm here with my little boy, Erkan. Our GP thought he might have asthma but he wasn't sure so he sent us here. I hope the doctor can find out what's wrong with him.

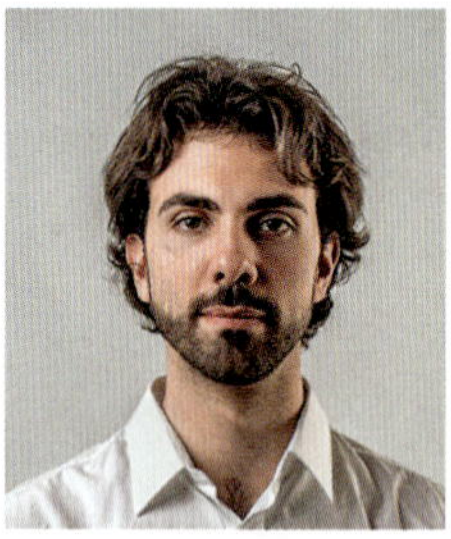

Andrew Carter
Well, I cut my arm while repairing a bike and it looked like a bad cut. This is the nearest health centre. It's really close by, so I walked here straightaway.

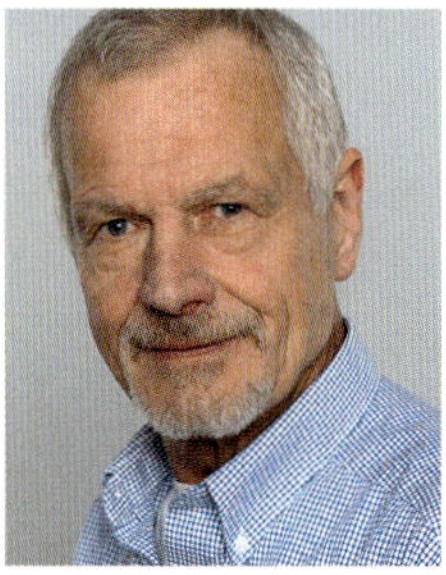

Ron Jarvis
Well, I'm a bit deaf at the moment, so I went to see the doctor last week and he told me it was just a problem with wax. So, I've got an appoint-ment today to have my ears syringed.

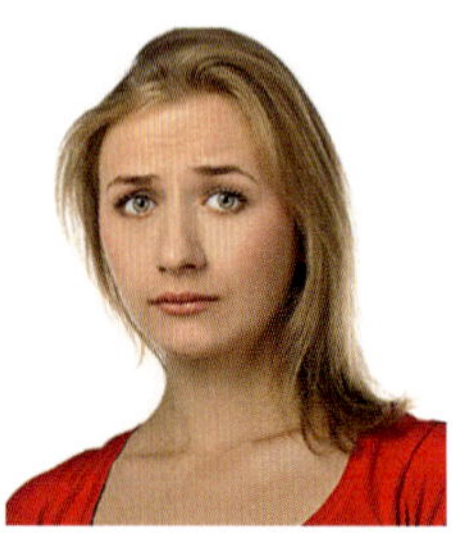

Karolina Bartolski
I'm here because I received a letter asking me to come for a smear test. It's only a routine test, but I think it's a really good idea to have regular check-ups.

2 Seeing the nurse

Sandra is a nurse at a health centre in the UK. She is syringing a patient's ear.

A 15 **Complete the dialogue with the simple past form of the verbs. Be careful of negatives and questions. Then listen to the CD to check your answers.**

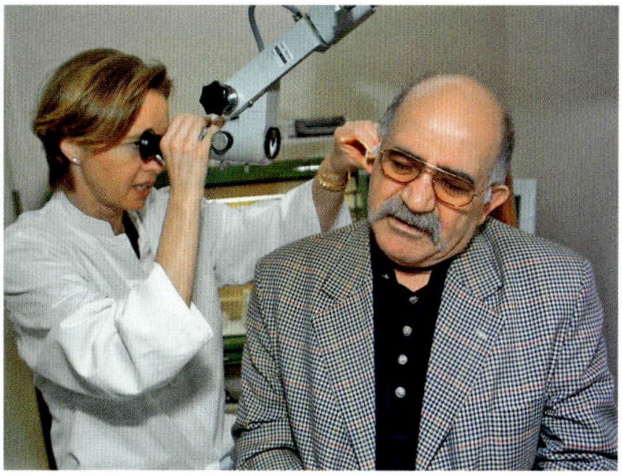

Sandra Hello, good morning Mr Jarvis. My name's Sandra Waterman. How are you today?

Ron Very well, thanks.

Sandra Is this your first visit to our practice?

Ron Yes, it is. I ___ (move)[1] to the town three months ago.

Sandra Oh really? And where ___ you ___ (live)[2] before?

Ron In a small village called Shepton, about six miles away.

Sandra Oh, I know Shepton very well. It's a pretty place, isn't it?

Ron Yes, it is. Very.

Sandra Now, can you hold this tray for me under your ear?

Ron Yes, I can, sure.

Sandra: That's great, thanks. And who ___ (be)[3] your GP there?

Ron I ___ (go)[4] to Dr Wheeler at the Maltings Health Centre.

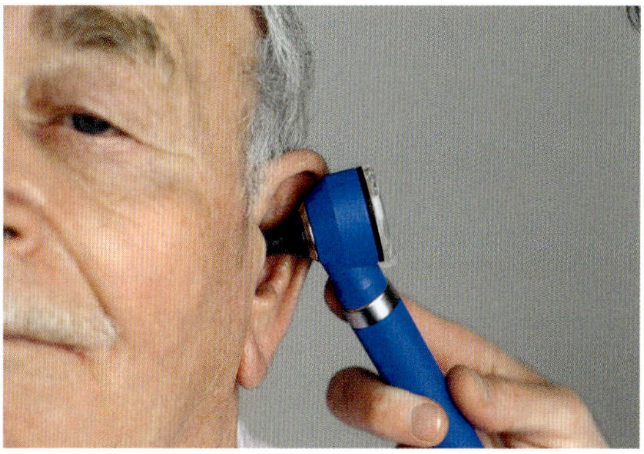

Sandra Oh yes, Dr Wheeler's very nice. I ___ (live)[5] in Shepton for five years, but I ___ (not/work)[6] at the Maltings.

Ron Where ___ you ___ (work)[7]?

Sandra I ___ (work)[8] here! Now I'm going to start syringing your ear. Tell me if it hurts at all, OK? Right, here we go. I moved here fifteen years ago but I ___ (begin)[9] working here twenty years ago.

Ron That's a long time! ___ you always ___ (want)[10] to be a nurse?

Sandra Yes, I did. I ___ (know)[11] I wanted to be a nurse when I ___ (be)[12] still at school.

Ron So, did you leave school and start your training straightaway?

Sandra Yes, I did. And then this ___ (be)[13] the first job I ___ (apply)[14] for. Is this comfortable for you? It isn't painful at all?

Ron No, it isn't, it's fine. I think I can hear better already!

B **Are the following statements true or false? Say why/why not.**

1 Mr Jarvis is a new patient.
2 Today, Sandra lives in the same village as Mr Jarvis.
3 Dr Wheeler is Mr Jarvis's doctor.
4 Sandra worked with Dr Wheeler.
5 Sandra lived in Shepton five years ago.
6 Sandra always wanted to be a nurse.
7 As soon as Sandra left school she began her training.
8 Ron said the syringing hurt a little.

Answering yes/no questions

1 **Is** this your first visit to our practice? Yes, it **is**.
2 **Is** it painful at all? No, it **isn't**.
3 **Are** you from Shepton? No, I'**m not**.
4 **Does** it hurt? No, it **doesn't**.
5 **Did** you always want to be a nurse? Yes, I **did**.

– *Yes/No* Antworten werden mit *yes/no*, einem Pronomen und demgleichen Hilfsverb oder Verb *to be* wie in der Frage gebildet. (1–5)

Common medical abbreviations

ENT	Ears, nose and throat
ECG	An electrocardiograph is a machine that measures the electrical charges in your heart.
EEG	An electroencephalograph is a machine that measures electrical activity in the brain.

3 Practice

Answer the following questions using a yes/no answer: answer four with yes and four with no.

1 Are you sitting comfortably?
2 Is she a registered patient?
3 Does that hurt?
4 Is this your home address?
5 Did you have to wait long?
6 Do you live near the practice?
7 Are the tests positive?
8 Did she make an appointment?

4 The nose, mouth and throat

A **16)) Listen to a GP talking to a class of trainee nurses about the nose, mouth and throat. Match the numbers in the diagram to the words below.**

gullet (oesophagus) · olfactory nerves · throat · windpipe (trachea) · palate · tongue · nasal passage

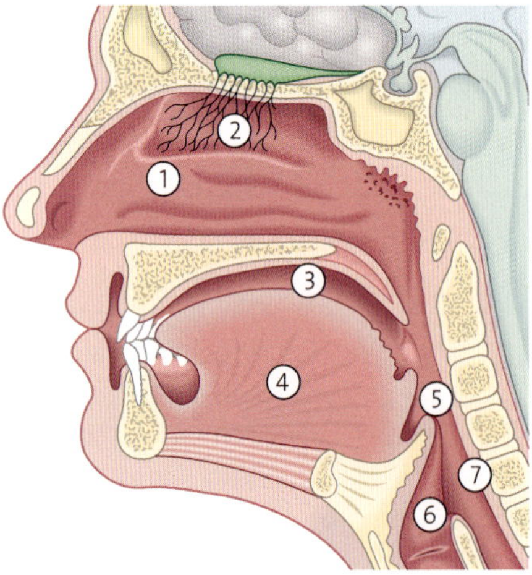

B **Listen again and, using the diagram, make notes to explain the function of the nose, mouth and throat.**

5 Working with words

Which parts of the nose and mouth do you use when you taste and smell?

6 Practice

Complete the sentences with a suitable preposition.

1 If you look ___ your books ___ page 32, you'll see the diagram ___ the nose, mouth and throat.
2 The nasal passage at the start ___ the nose takes air ___ the body.
3 The air goes ___ the nasal passage and then it passes ___ the olfactory nerves.
4 These nerves send information about smell all the way ___ the brain.
5 The air then goes down into the back of the mouth and ___ the trachea or windpipe.
6 ___ the middle of the mouth we can see the palate, which is the roof ___ the mouth.
7 When we eat or drink, food goes ___ the mouth into the back ___ our throats.
8 And when we swallow, food goes ___ our gullet and ___ there into the stomach.

7 Making a diagnosis

Bekri Özalan goes to see Dr Müller with a sore throat.

Copy the table below into your exercise book. Then read the text and complete the notes.

Patient	*Mr Bekri Özalan*
Symptoms	
Diagnosis	
Treatment	

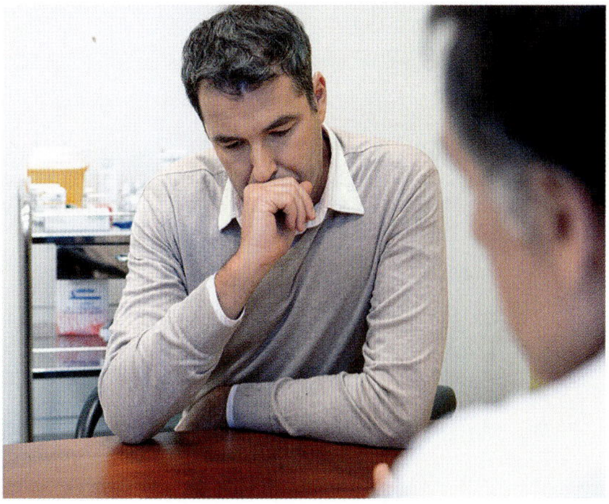

Dr Müller Good morning, Mr Özalan. Please come in. Now, tell me, what's the problem?

Bekri Özalan My throat is very sore and I'm not feeling very well.

Dr Müller OK, let's have a look. Can you please put your head back and open your mouth nice and wide? Thank you. Hmm. When did your throat start feeling sore?

Bekri Özalan About two days ago. It's really sore this morning actually. I'm also having trouble swallowing.

Dr Müller Uh huh. Can I take a quick look in your ears for a moment, please? Right, that looks OK. Now I just need to put this thermometer in your ear to take your temperature. There we go. Is that OK?

Bekri Özalan Yes, that's OK.

Dr Müller Right, your temperature is a little high. I just need to check your glands now. Hmm, they also feel a bit swollen. Are you having any problems breathing at all?

Bekri Özalan No, breathing is OK, but I can't sleep very well and I feel tired all the time.

Dr Müller Well, Mr Özalan, you have a temperature, your glands are a little swollen and your tonsils are also inflamed, so I think you probably have tonsillitis. I'd like to take a throat swab and send it to a lab to find out what caused the infection.

Bekri Özalan OK.

Dr Müller Can you open wide, please, so I can take a swab? That's it. Thank you. I'll send this to the lab for tests.

Bekri Özalan How long does that normally take?

Dr Müller Only a couple of days. They are pretty quick.

Bekri Özalan That's good.

Dr Müller To be on the safe side, I would like to prescribe some antibiotics. Are you allergic to any antibiotics?

Bekri Özalan No, not as far as I know.

Dr Müller Good. Well, take the tablets three times a day after meals, OK? And drink plenty of fluids, get some rest and come back in two days. I'll write you a sick note. OK?

Bekri Özalan Yes, thank you, doctor.

Dr Müller You're welcome. See you on Wednesday then.

LANGUAGE

Asking about symptoms
Could you tell me what's wrong?
What seems to be the problem?
Do you have/Have you got ...?
Does your neck/back/... hurt/ache?
When did this / the pain / the problem / ... start?
How long have you had this problem / this sore ...?

8 Working with words

A Match the verb phrases with the nouns.

1	take somebody's	a	tests
2	check somebody's	b	temperature
3	cause an	c	antibiotics
4	send for	d	fluids
5	prescribe	e	glands
6	drink plenty of	f	infection

B Then write a sentence with each matched verb phrase and noun.

9 What seems to be the problem?

These patients are waiting to see Dr Scott at a health centre in Britain.

A Write their names in a table in your exercise book.

Names	Symptoms

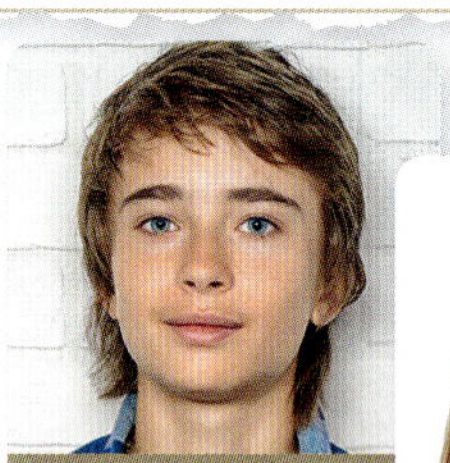
Stephen Carr

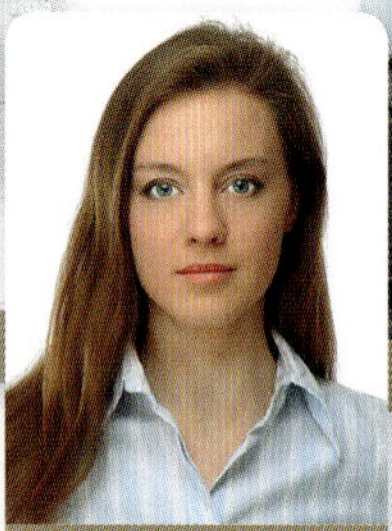
Cindy Taylor

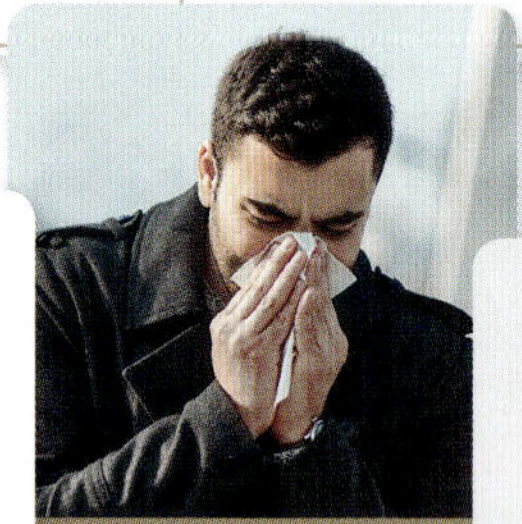
Özden Tuncay

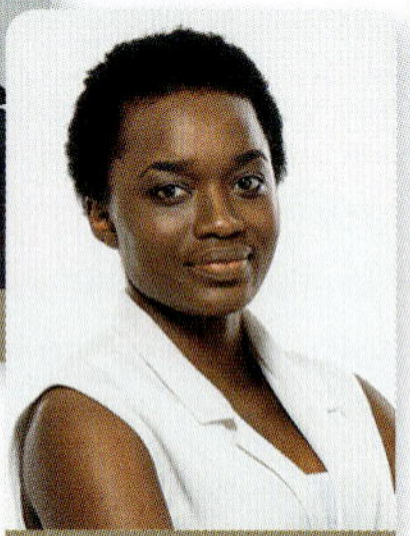
Mary Anderson

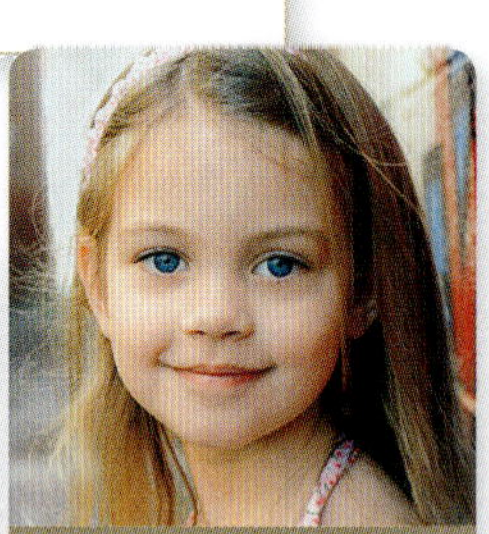
Lucy Morris

B 17)) Now listen to these patients or their parents talking to Dr Scott. Write down their symptoms.

10 Your diagnosis

Work with a partner and discuss each of the patients from exercise 9 and their symptoms. What is your diagnosis?

I think ___ has got ___ a cold.
food poisoning.
the flu.
an ear infection.
(the) measles.

I agree (with you / your diagnosis). I disagree. He/She could have ___ .

The symptoms for ___ are similar / different.

11 Examining the patient

Dr Scott is now ready to see Andrew Carter.

A 18 Listen and note down the details.

B Work with a partner and take turns asking and answering questions.

When Where What How	did	Mr Carter Dr Scott	cut his arm? treat him? give him? …?

12 Working with words

Copy and complete the table with the correct form of the words.

	verb	noun
1	diagnose	
2		examination
3	treat	
4	cut	
5	consult	
6	stitch	
7		look
8		dressing

LANGUAGE

Describing symptoms

I have / I've got
- a headache / a sore throat.
- backache / stomach ache / earache.
- chest/back/stomach pains.
- a pain in my …

I keep coughing/sneezing/vomiting.
I have trouble sleeping / breathing / keeping food down / …
My joints/feet/head ache(s).

13 Describing symptoms

Work with a partner. One student thinks of a medical problem and describes the typical symptoms. The other guesses what the problem is by asking questions.

Have you got a sore throat?	No, I haven't.
Have you got a temperature?	Yes, I have.
Do your joints ache?	Yes, they do.

14 Mediation: B1

Situation: In Ihrer Praxis gibt es ein recht unübersichtliches Merkblatt für die Mitarbeiter, was bei der Untersuchung von Patienten generell zu beachten ist. Da in letzter Zeit immer mehr Patienten zu Ihnen kommen, mit denen Sie auf Englisch kommunizieren müssen, soll ein Leitfaden erstellt werden, der in englischer Sprache auflistet, was in welcher Reihenfolge zu tun ist. Die behandelnden Ärzte gehen davon aus, dass ein solcher Leitfaden auch ihnen die Kommunikation erleichtert.
→ **Übertragen Sie die Aussagen des deutschen Merkblatts für einen Leitfaden in englischer Sprache. Dieser soll in knapper Form Anweisungen enthalten. Nummerieren Sie diese.**

Das **Merkblatt** hat folgenden Wortlaut:

Falls der Patient / die Patientin Sie noch nie gesehen hat, sollten Sie sich zunächst vorstellen. Sie dürfen ein paar freundliche Worte wechseln, um für eine entspannte Atmosphäre zu sorgen. Messen Sie den Puls und den Blutdruck und notieren Sie beide. Lassen Sie sich die Beschwerden erklären. Bitten Sie den Patienten / die Patientin, sich hinzulegen oder hinzusetzen und die Kleidung für den betreffenden Körperteil zu entfernen.

Sagen Sie stets, was Sie vorhaben, bevor Sie den Patienten / die Patientin berühren. Erwähnen Sie ggf. auch, welche Instrumente Sie dafür benutzen und welche Wirkung sie haben könnten. Vergessen Sie nicht, den Patienten / die Patientin immer wieder zu beruhigen. Auch Lächeln schafft Vertrauen! Wenn Sie untersuchen, fragen Sie immer wieder, ob es weh tut und auch wo genau. Beachten Sie stets die Hygienevorschriften! Am Ende Ihrer Untersuchung fassen Sie das Ergebnis zusammen und erklären, welche Maßnahmen / Schritte erforderlich sind. Verabschieden Sie sich beim Patienten / bei der Patientin mit seinem / ihrem Namen und wünschen ihm / ihr gute Besserung.

15 Produktion: B1

Situation: Nachdem der Leitfaden in englischer Sprache angefertigt wurde, soll dieser für bestimmte, häufig vorkommende Untersuchungen konkretisiert werden.
→ **Passen Sie den Leitfaden an eine der folgenden Untersuchungen an:**

- a **Ultraschalluntersuchung der Nieren,**
- b **Bauchschmerzen,**
- c **Halsschmerzen bei einer fiebrigen Erkältung,**
- d **Atembeschwerden oder**
- e **Gelenkbeschwerden im Knie,**

am besten entsprechend der Fachrichtung, für die Sie tätig sind.
Falls Sie eine Berechtigung zum Röntgen besitzen, erwähnen Sie auch die hierfür erforderlichen Schritte.

16 Women and heart disease

A Read the article about heart disease and answer the questions below.

My 'flu' was a heart attack!

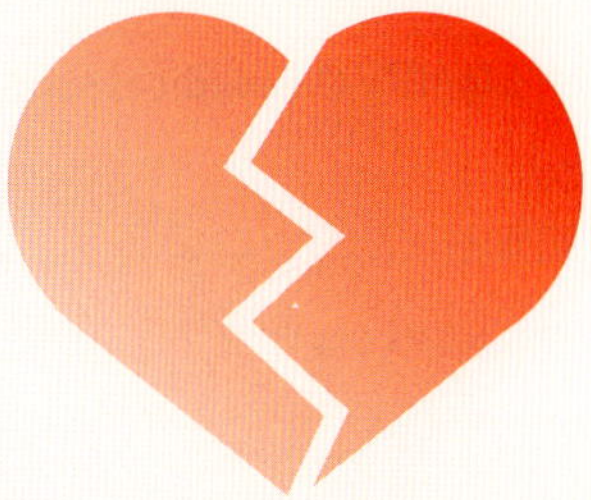

More women than men in Europe die from heart disease, but many still don't recognize the symptoms. The warning signs could be very different to those for men, as Alison Morgan found out …

When we think of heart disease, we think of middle-aged men who are overweight and under stress at work. But across Europe, 55 per cent of women now die from heart disease compared with 43 per cent of men.

Alison was only 40 when she had a mild heart attack last year. "I was at work, running up some stairs after smoking a cigarette," she says. "When I got to the top of the stairs, I couldn't breathe. I felt dizzy and weak. I had a headache and it felt like flu symptoms. I didn't have any chest pains."

Alison went to see her GP who also first thought she had flu symptoms. However, when the doctor took Alison's pulse, it was above the normal heart rate. She carried out an ECG test and told Alison it was a heart attack. "An ambulance was called straightaway and my doctor told me to stay calm."

"Women still have the view that it's a man's disease," says Dr Colin Anderson, consultant cardiologist and medical director of the British Heart Foundation. "I think there are a number of reasons for that – it's mainly much older women who have coronary heart disease, and people still believe that heart attacks happen to stressed, over-worked men. But, of course, women are dealing with stress in their lives too, and another problem is that quite a high number of women smoke."

Although several traditional risk factors such as high blood pressure, smoking and obesity affect men and women, there are additional factors that play a bigger role in the development of heart disease in women. Women with diabetes, for example, are at a greater risk than men. We also know that women's hearts are affected by depression more than men's. Finally, the menopause – the low levels of oestrogen after menopause present a significant risk factor for developing cardiovascular disease.

1 Describe the typical 'heart attack candidate'.
2 Why didn't Alison think she had heart disease?
3 What causes might there be for Alison's heart disease?

B Use the information given in the text to design a leaflet for your German patients and make sure you include the typical warning signals.

5 Treating a patient

1 Surgery equipment

Here are some typical medical supplies that a medical assistant works with.

A Identify the medical supplies and equipment in the photos below.

examination gloves · hypodermic (syringe) · disinfectant · elastic bandage · thermometer · tourniquet · (a pair of) tweezers · (a pair of) scissors · gauze dressing · (cotton) swabs · scalpel · stethoscope · otoscope · blood-pressure cuff · surgical needle-holder · needle-thread combination

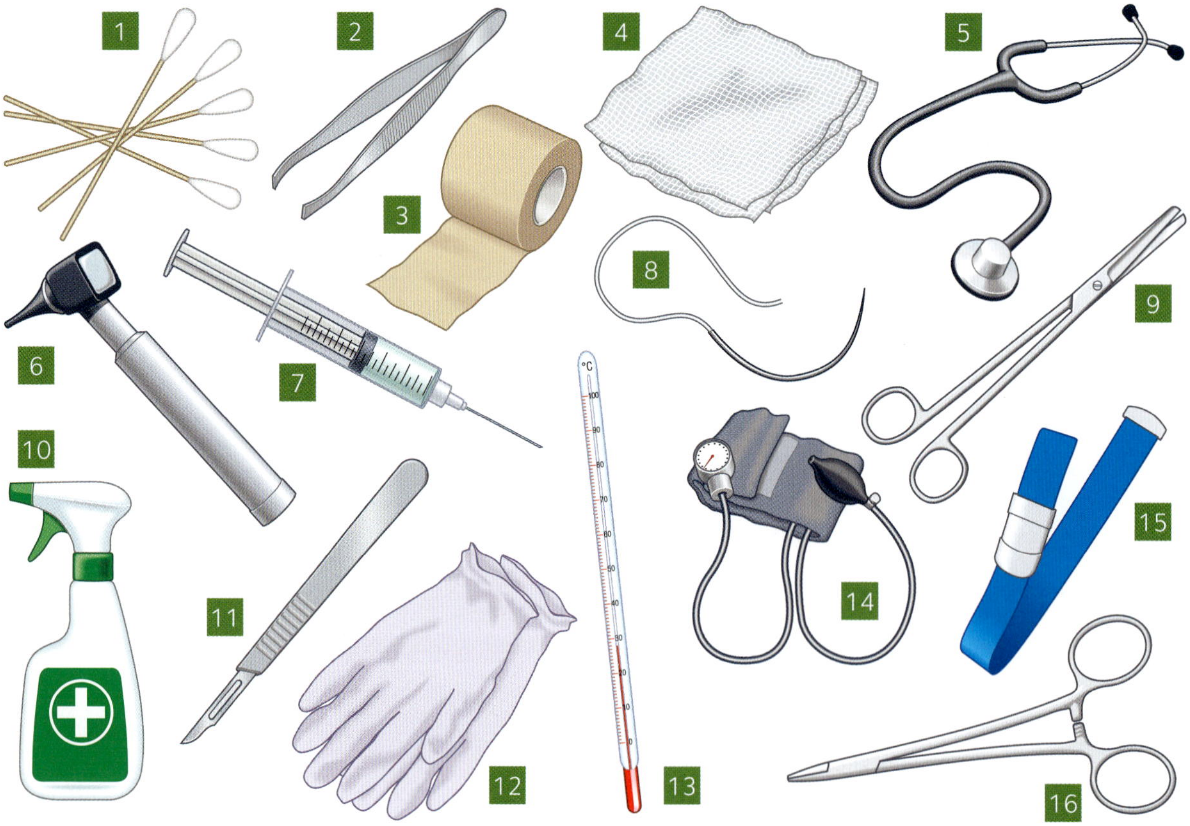

B **Work with a partner. Use the words below to describe what each piece of equipment is used for.**

> A thermometer is used to take a patient's temperature.

> Swabs are used to clean wounds.

> You use a gauze dressing to dress a wound.

take · give · clean · cut · stitch · dress · examine · extract · listen to · inject · protect · measure

a wound · a dressing · a cut · blood · patients · the heartbeat · a patient's temperature · an injection · a sprain · ears · blood pressure · splinters · the skin · broken glass · hands

2 Stitching a wound

Dr Müller and Kerstin are treating a deep cut on a patient's arm at their health centre in Passau.

A **Describe what they are doing in each step and name the instruments they are using.**

give local anaesthetic · take stitches out · examine wound · tie off stitches · clean wound · dress wound · stitch wound

LANGUAGE

Sequence words
First … | Then … | Next … | After that … | Finally …

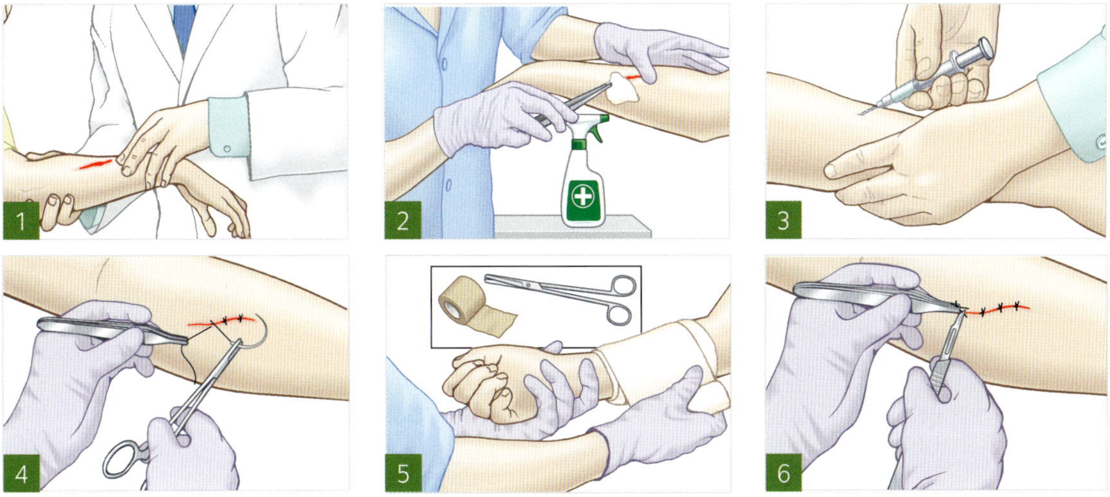

Ten days later

First
Then
Next
After that
Finally

B 19 **Now listen and check your answers.**

C Now complete the dialogue with the correct form of the present continuous.

Dr Müller So, Mr Gray, this is going to sting a bit.

Mr Gray Ouch!

Dr Müller I ___ (just/clean)[1] the wound before I start stitching. That all looks good – nice and clean. Do you have the hypodermic, please, Kerstin? Thanks. I ___ (give)[2] you a local anaesthetic now, Mr Gray, so you won't feel the stitches.

Mr Gray OK, thanks.

Dr Müller It'll take a minute or two for the anaesthetic to take effect. I'll be back in a moment.
Hello again, Mr Gray, how ___ (you/do)[3]? While Kerstin ___ (get)[4] everything ready, I'm going to just clean the wound again. There we are. Ready?

Mr Gray Yes.

Dr Müller Good. If you wish, you can look away while I ___ (do)[5] the stitches.

Mr Gray That's a good idea. I think I will.

Dr Müller No problem. I ___ (just/start)[6] the first stitch now. It doesn't hurt, does it?

Mr Gray No. I can feel that you ___ (do)[7] the stitches, but it doesn't hurt.

Dr Müller That's good. Nearly there. I ___ (just/finish)[8] off the last one. And now I ___ (tie off)[9] the stitches. There we are. Kerstin, could you please dress the wound? Thank you.

Kerstin OK, Mr Gray, this won't take very long. There we are, nearly done. I think it's safe for you to look again.

Mr Gray OK, thanks.

Dr Müller I'll leave Kerstin to finish off, and we'll see you in a few days.

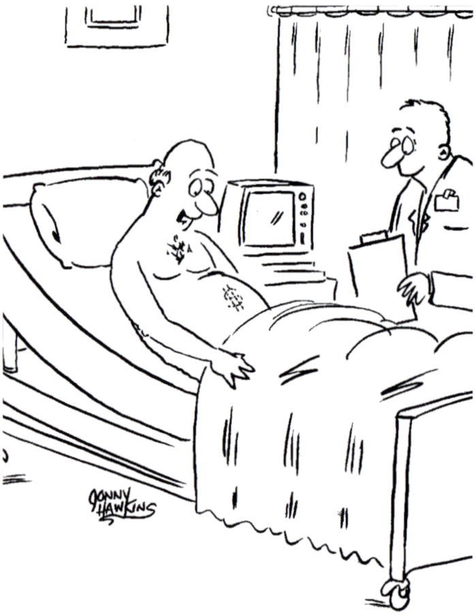

"Nice stitches, Doc."

Present continuous (Verlaufsform der Gegenwart)

1. **I'm tying off** the stitches now.
2. Kerstin **is getting** the treatment room ready for Dr Müller.
3. **I'm not working** here permanently.
4. Dr Müller's colleague is on holiday and **is returning** in five days.
5. What **are** you **doing** this evening?

- Das *present continuous* beschreibt Ereignisse oder Aktionen, die gerade passieren (1, 2) oder kurzfristige Situation, die sich bald ändern. (3)
- Das *present continuous* wird für festgelegte Vereinbarungen in der Zukunft verwendet. (4, 5)
- Typische Signalwörter sind: *now, at the moment, just.*
- Das *present continuous* wird mit *am/is/are* + *-ing*-Form gebildet. (1–5)
- Die Verneinung wird mit *am not (I'm not) /isn't/aren't* gebildet. (3)
- Um Fragen zu bilden, vertauscht man *am/is/are* mit dem Subjekt. (5)

3 Practice

Make questions using the present continuous.

1 How many patients ___ ___ to see Dr Carey? (wait)
2 Which patient ___ Dr Kingsley ___ now? (treat)
3 ___ you still ___ unwell, Mrs Enderby? (feel)
4 ___ this medication ___ the pain, Mr Jones? (stop)
5 Caroline, ___ you ___ everything ready for the stitching procedure? (get)
6 ___ Dr Müller ___ Mr Gray at the moment? (treat)
7 ___ the anaesthetic ___? (work)
8 ___ Mr and Mrs Appleby ___ the doctor right now? (see)

4 Taking blood

Mary Smith is one of Dr Müller's patients. She has got an appointment for an immunization. Before the doctor gives Mary the injection, she asks Kerstin to do a blood test.

Look at the illustrations and role-play the dialogue between Mary and Kerstin.

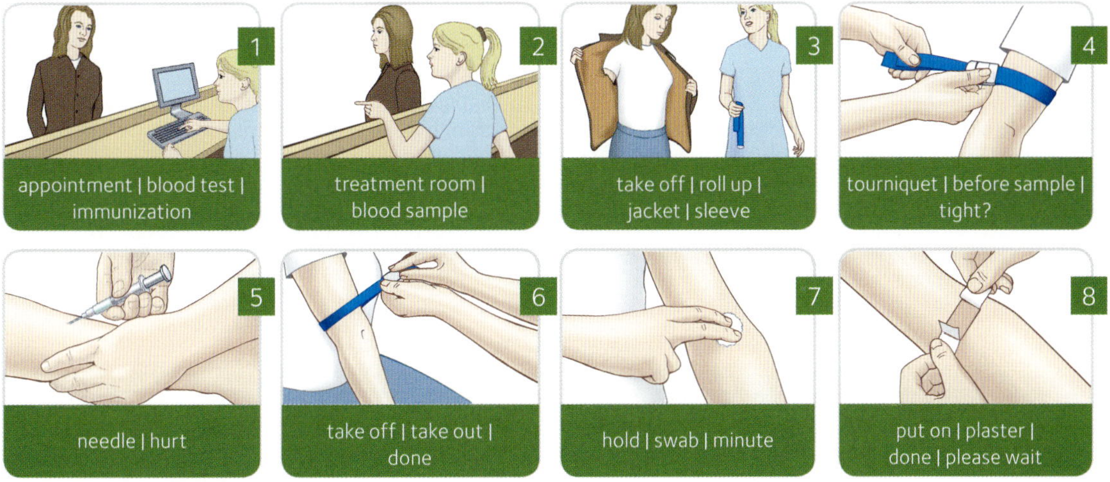

20))) Now listen to the actual dialogue and compare with your versions.

5 Practice

Complete the sentences with the correct preposition.

1 Good morning, I'm here for an immunization ___ hepatitis A.
2 Could you please wait ___ the doctor in the waiting room?
3 Please take ___ your jacket.
4 Can I ask you to roll ___ your sleeve, please?
5 First, we put ___ a tourniquet.
6 I'm just taking ___ the needle. There we are. All done.
7 Could you hold the swab ___ your arm for a minute?
8 And finally, just let me put a small plaster ___ your arm, OK?

6 Blood pressure

Medical assistants often take blood pressure and have to explain to a patient what the reading means.

Read the text and answer the patient's questions below.

How to read blood pressure numbers

Every time your heart beats your blood pressure first rises and then, when your heart relaxes between beats, it falls. So when we record blood pressure, we record two numbers, written like this:

$$\frac{117}{76}\ \text{mm Hg.}$$

We read the numbers as "117 over 76 (millimeters of mercury (Hg))". The top number measures the pressure in the arteries when the heart beats (when the heart muscle contracts). This is the 'systolic' pressure. The bottom number measures the pressure in the arteries between heartbeats (when the heart muscle is resting or relaxing). This is the 'diastolic' pressure. In most people, systolic blood pressure rises steadily with age due to increasing stiffness of large arteries, long-term build-up of plaque, and more frequent cardiac and vascular disease.

While blood pressure can change from minute to minute with changes in exercise, stress or sleep, it should normally be less than 120/80 mm Hg (less than 120 systolic AND less than 80 diastolic) for an adult aged 20 or over. If your blood pressure reading is higher than normal, your doctor may take several readings over time and/or ask you to monitor your blood pressure at home before diagnosing you with high blood pressure.

A single high reading does not necessarily mean that you have high blood pressure. However, if readings stay at 140/90 mm Hg or above over time, your doctor will likely want you to begin a treatment program. Such a program almost always includes lifestyle changes and often prescription medication for those with readings of 140/90 or higher.

If, while monitoring your blood pressure, you get repeated readings of 180 mm Hg or higher systolic or 110 mm Hg or higher diastolic pressure, you should seek immediate emergency medical treatment for a hypertensive crisis. If you can't get emergency medical help, ask someone to drive you to hospital straightaway.

Blood pressure category	Systolic (upper value) mm Hg	Diastolic (lower value) mm Hg
Low	70–89	less than 60
Normal	90–119	60–79
Prehypertension	120–139	80–89
High: Hypertension Stage 1	140–159	90–99
High: Hypertension Stage 2	160–179	100–109
High: Hypertension Stage 3 (crisis)	180–	110–

Why are there two numbers?

What's normal blood pressure?

Does age make a difference to blood pressure?

If I get a high reading, what do I do?

At what point would I need to start treatment?

If my blood pressure is extremely high, what do I need to do?

7 How to take blood pressure

Apparatus for a blood pressure test

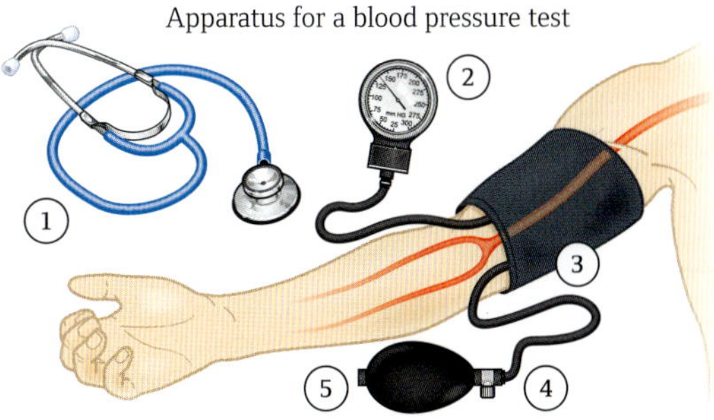

Kerstin is taking a patient's blood pressure.

A Match the names of the equipment to the numbers in the illustration.

bulb · cuff · gauge · stethoscope · valve

B Put the following steps in the correct order.

- a **Listen for the diastolic reading:** Continue to deflate the cuff until the sounds fade. The reading on the gauge when the sounds stop is the diastolic pressure.
- b **Double-check for accuracy:** Wait 5 mins. between readings. If the pressure is high, take further readings.
- c **Place the cuff on the patient's arm:** Locate the brachial artery and make sure the cuff fits snugly around the arm.
- d **Inflate the cuff:** Begin pumping the bulb until you stop the blood flow. You should hear no sounds through the stethoscope.
- e **Prepare the patient:** Make sure the patient is relaxed by allowing 5 minutes to relax before the first reading. Make sure no clothing gets in the way of the cuff. Ask the patient not to talk.
- f **Position the stethoscope:** On the same arm you put the cuff, locate a strong pulse and place the stethoscope over the brachial artery.
- g **Slowly deflate the cuff:** Open the valve to deflate the cuff until you hear a pulse. The first sounds you hear is the patient's systolic pressure.

8 Taking a patient's blood pressure

Work with a partner to make a dialogue.

Medical assistant

Begrüßen Sie den Patient / die Patientin. Bitten Sie ihn/sie, den Ärmel hoch zu krempeln.

Patient

Fragen Sie, ob es so in Ordnung ist.

Medical assistant

Bejahen Sie. Erklären Sie, dass Sie zunächst den Blutdruck messen werden. Fragen Sie, ob es dem Patienten / der Patientin gut geht.

Patient

Bestätigen Sie, dass alles bestens ist.

Medical assistant

Teilen Sie dem Patienten / der Patientin den Blutdruckwert mit: 150/90 mm Hg.

Patient

Bitten Sie die MFA um Erklärung, ob der Wert in Ordnung ist. Fragen Sie, was die beiden Zahlen bedeuten.

Medical assistant

Erklären Sie die Zahlen. Sagen Sie, dass die Werte etwas hoch sind und Sie den Blutdruck noch einmal messen möchten.

Patient

Fragen Sie, was der Normalwert ist.

Medical assistant

Sagen Sie, was der Normalwert ist und beruhigen Sie den Patienten / die Patientin.

9 Leseverstehen

Situation: Sie sind mit einer deutschen Touristengruppe in England. Eine schwangere Mitreisende hat in der Freiwahl einer Drogerie, in der es auch eine Abteilung für verschreibungspflichtige Medikamente gibt, ein Nahrungsergänzungsmittel, dessen Hauptbestandteile Cranberries sind, gekauft, weil man ihr wegen ihrer Blasenschwäche dazu geraten hatte. Sie präsentiert Ihnen das beliegende Informationsblatt und bittet Sie, ihr in Kürze (auch stichwortartig) aufzuschreiben, ob sie als Schwangere besondere Hinweise zu beachten habe und welche Nebenwirkungen sich ergeben könnten.

→ Erstellen Sie für die Mitreisende Hinweise mit den gewünschten Informationen in deutscher Sprache. Lesen Sie dafür den Text des Beipackzettels genau durch. Ihre schriftlichen Hinweise sind knapp und übersichtlich.

Cranberry is used for:

Urinary tract infections, to decrease odour from loss of bladder control (incontinence), and for kidney stones. Cranberry is a herbal product. It contains a substance that blocks bacteria from attaching to the bladder wall.

Do NOT use cranberry if you are allergic to any ingredient in cranberry.

Before using cranberry:

Some medical conditions may interact with cranberry. Tell your doctor or pharmacist if you have any medical conditions, especially if any of the following apply to you:

- if you are pregnant, planning to become pregnant, or are breast-feeding
- if you are currently taking any prescription or nonprescription medicine, herbal preparation, or dietary supplement
- if you have diabetes or a history of kidney stones

How to use cranberry:

Use cranberry as directed by your doctor and check the label on the medicine for exact dosing instructions.

- Cranberry may be taken as juice or as capsules or tablets containing the dried cranberry powder.
- Drinking extra fluids while you are taking this product is recommended.
- If you miss taking a dose of cranberry for one or more days, there is no cause for concern. If your doctor recommended that you take it, try to remember your dose every day.

Important safety information:

This product has not been approved by the Food and Drug Administration (FDA) as safe and effective for any medical condition. The long-term safety of herbal products is not known. Before using any alternative medicine, talk with your doctor or pharmacist.

PREGNANCY and BREAST-FEEDING: If you plan on becoming pregnant, discuss with your doctor the benefits and risks of using this product during pregnancy. If you are or will be breast-feeding while you are using this product, check with your doctor or pharmacist to discuss the risks to your baby.

Possible side effects of cranberry:

All medicines may cause side effects, but many people have no, or minor, side effects. No COMMON side effects have been reported with the proper use of cranberry. Seek medical attention right away if any of these SEVERE side effects occur:

Severe allergic reactions are possible (rash; hives; itching; difficulty breathing; tightness in the chest; swelling of the mouth, face, lips, or tongue).

This is not a complete list of all the side effects that may occur. If you have questions about side effects, contact your healthcare provider. Call your doctor for medical advice about side effects.

10 Video conferencing

Your boss is thinking about using video conferencing at your health centre. He has asked you to find out about it. You find this text on the internet.

The future of remote medical consultations

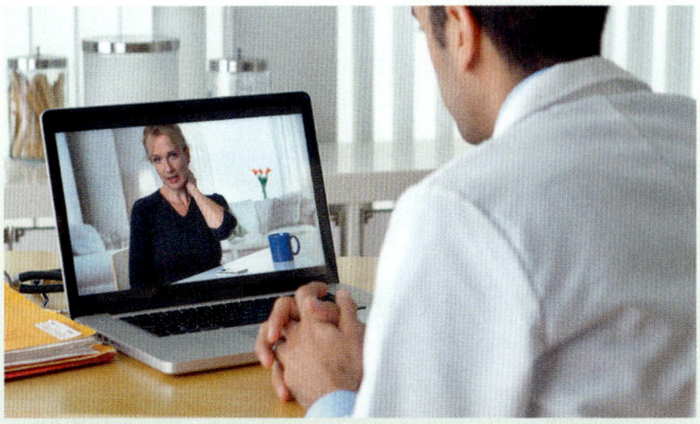

Connecting doctors with patients by video is not new – but is now the time for it to finally take off?

Aberdeen Royal Infirmary in Scotland is conducting an experiment in telemedicine – diagnosing and treating medical conditions by video conferencing. The trial is to check whether teleconsultations are as good as face-to-face ones.

The technology is a video conferencing system which presents a life-size, high-definition image of the patient as if they were sitting just across the table. The patient's booth includes medical devices – such as a stethoscope, blood-pressure cuff and thermometer – to send important information to the doctor. The whole setup works on a standard broadband network and the experience is very close to life. "It was just like a normal consultation," says a patient.

Patients who volunteer for teleconsultations also have face-to-face examinations. The next stage will be to move the patient booth to a "remote safe site", probably a community hospital, where hands-on medical help is available. If that works, the booth could go almost anywhere – maybe even to a hotel or a police station.

Even if the trials succeed, creating a full service may be difficult. Setting up a sponsored pilot trial is one thing, running an ongoing service across the whole NHS is quite another. The lesson of 50 years of telemedicine is that, even if the technology can work, it is only one part of a much larger jigsaw puzzle.

A Are the statements below true or false? Correct the false statements.

1 The trials are taking place in three UK hospitals.
2 The trial is to see how good the face-to-face consultations are.
3 There is medical equipment in the patient booth.
4 The system uses special network technology.
5 Patients in the trial also have face-to-face consultations.
6 The booths will only be used in hospitals.
7 If the trial is successful, booths will be used all over the UK.

B Your boss now asks you for a recommendation about whether it is a good idea or not for the health centre.

Give as many advantages and disadvantages as you can think of.

6 Dealing with anxious patients

1 Understanding patient needs

These people are in the waiting room of your practice.

A 21 Listen and find out who they are and why they are there.

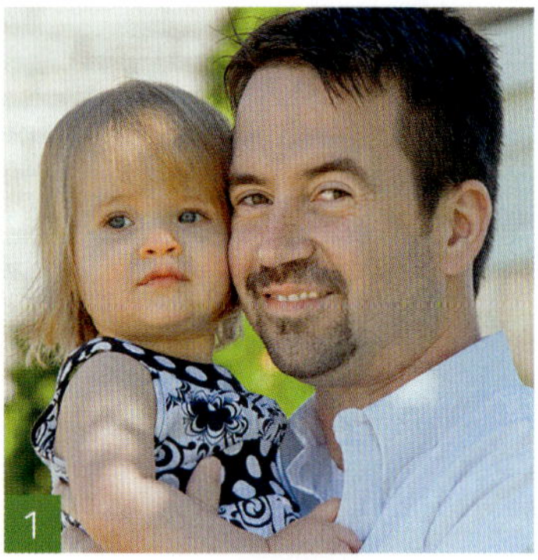

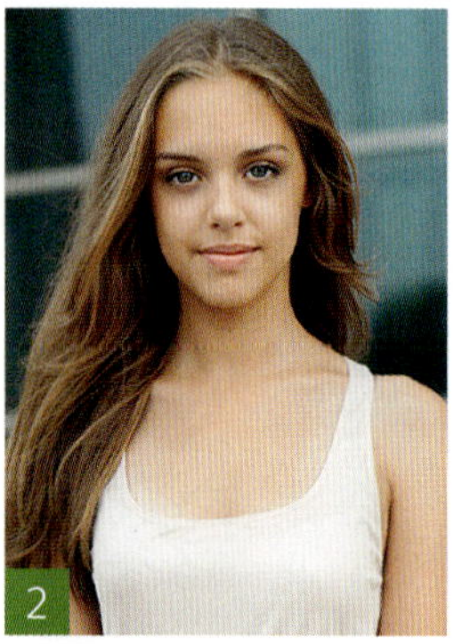

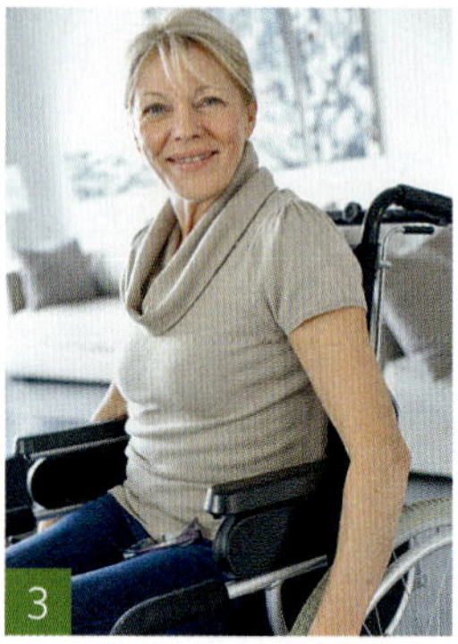

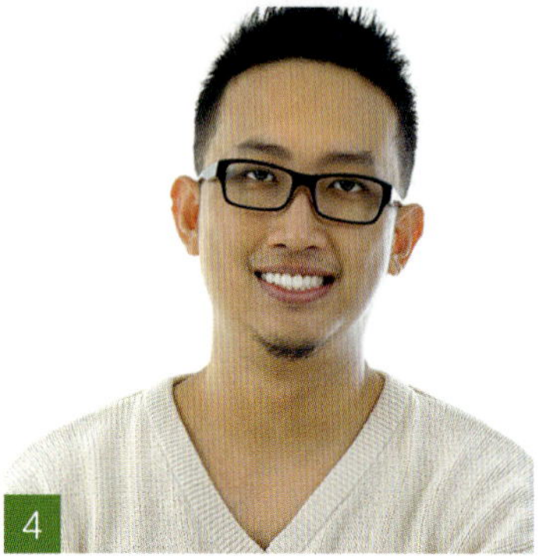

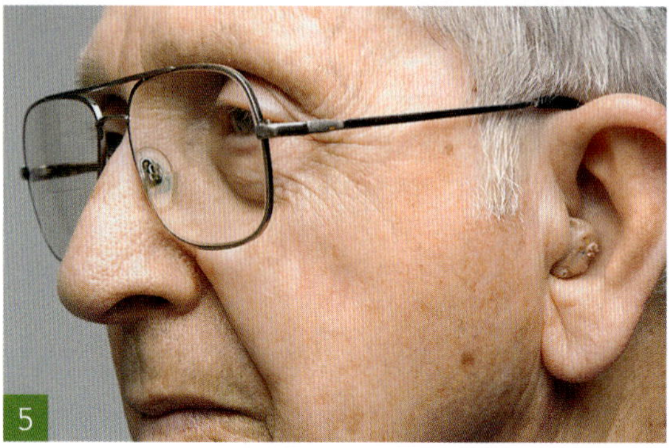

Photo 1 shows ___

Barney · Mike · Li · Rachel · Shelley · Susan

back pain · blood and urine samples · pelvic examination · prescription medication · smallpox vaccination · tetanus injection

B Which word is the odd one out? Give a reason for your choice.

1	a injection	b medication	c sample	d prescription
2	a awful	b bad	c serious	d coughing
3	a nervous	b anxious	c pain	d scared

C What special needs do you think the patients on page 46 might have? Think about health problems, language difficulties, cultural differences, physical and mental needs. Make suggestions about how you could help them.

I notice that ▬ needs/has got a	hearing aid. wheelchair. pushchair. Chinese name. ▬	

He/She	is looks seems must be	disabled. partially deaf. anxious. nervous. ▬

I	can could	give ▬ bring ▬ help ▬ with help ▬ to take ▬ to speak ▬	a toy. a magazine. getting out of ▬. undress. the toilet. an explanation. slowly/clearly. ▬

2 What makes us anxious?

Everyone feels anxious sometimes. How anxious do the following situations make you feel?

Work with a partner. Rate them on a scale of 1 to 5 (1 = relaxed, 2 = nervous, 3 = tense, 4 = worried, 5 = very anxious).

a speaking English
b having dental treatment
c taking an English exam
d travelling by plane
e a job interview
f having an injection

LANGUAGE

Expressing anxiety
I'm afraid of / scared of / anxious about …
… makes me nervous / feel uncomfortable.
I worry about …

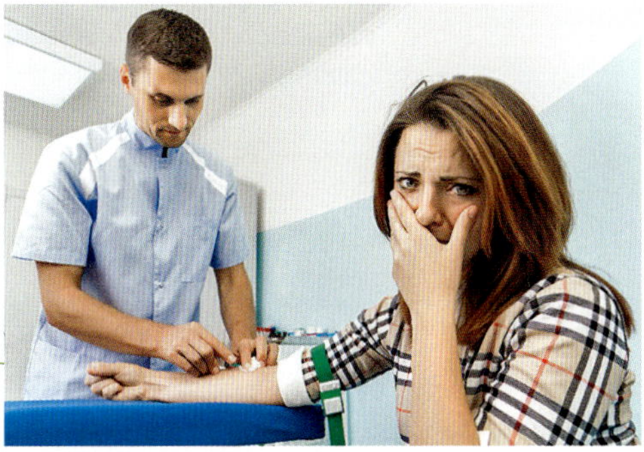

3 Patient anxiety

Read the text on the next page and match the paragraphs with the headings below.

a Fear of physical pain
b No news is good news
c Anxiety about illness and death
d Poor communication skills
e Fear of infection

Are you anxious in the doctor's practice?

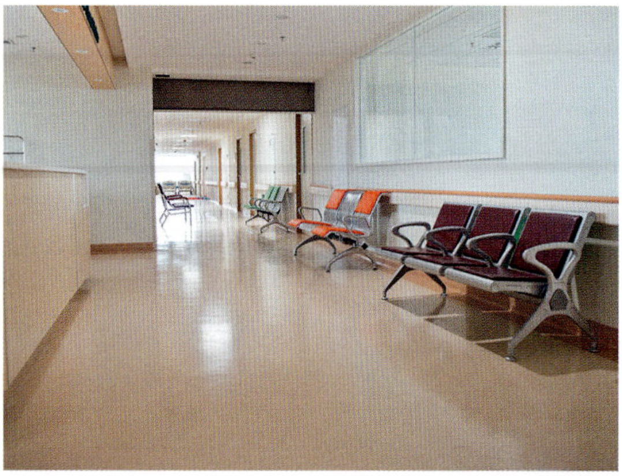

Millions of people hate visiting the doctor. They are often afraid of visiting the doctor's practice or a hospital because such places have a certain smell and atmosphere to them. They can smell of medicine and that can be scary for some people.

1 Another common cause of anxiety is the fact that a doctor's practice and a hospital are where people are sick and suffering from diseases such as cancer and other life-threatening conditions. Some people are uncomfortable when around others who are seriously ill.

2 Many people are scared of doctors themselves. Doctors often have a certain kind of 'coldness' to them. They are trained to be objective, which can make them seem 'distant' and 'cold'. When doctors are 'cold' and don't seem friendly, patients can feel as if they are just a number on a sheet of paper.

3 A lot of people are scared of the doctor because they associate the doctor with painful things, such as injections and needles. People often don't understand what their treatment involves and so feel helpless because they have no control over what is going to happen.

4 Also, doctors can find out scary things about us. We often go to see our doctor with symptoms but no idea about the cause. Sometimes, a doctor may give us bad news and we are afraid that there is something very seriously wrong with us. Many people would rather not hear the truth.

5 Many people think going to the doctor or visiting a hospital is a health risk. They think that places full of sick people are also full of germs and they are worried about catching something and becoming sicker than when they went in.

4 True or false?

Read the text again and say whether the following statements are true or false. Correct the false statements in your exercise book.

1 Not many people worry about going to the doctor's practice.
2 A cool, clinical atmosphere makes patients feel comfortable.
3 A lot of people don't like being around other sick people.
4 Doctors are trained to be cold and unfriendly.
5 Fear of pain is another common reason for being nervous.
6 Patients don't want the doctor to explain the treatment to them.
7 When people don't know what's wrong with them, they fear the worst.
8 Some patients think they will get germs from visiting the practice.

5 How to deal with anxiety

Look at the list of ways of dealing with patient anxiety.

Which treatments/procedures would be useful for an anxious patient? Give reasons. Does your surgery offer any of these? If so, which? If you are involved, what is your role?

a relaxing music
b general anaesthetic
c listening to the patient
d watching TV during treatment
e explaining the treatment fully
f using modern instruments
g a relaxing foot spa
h relaxing atmosphere in the surgery
i massaging the patient
j aromatherapy candles
k toys for children, children's corner

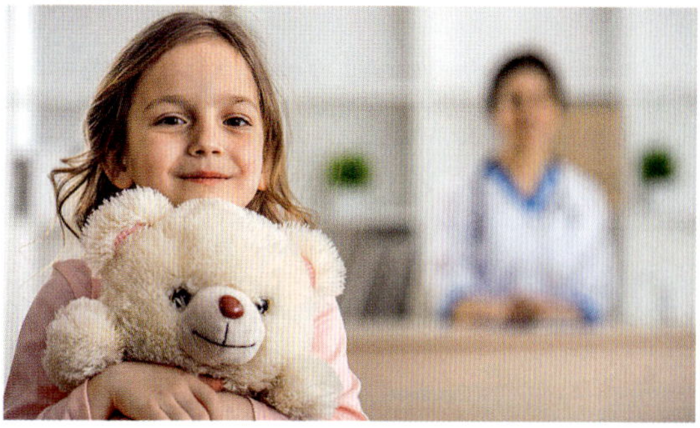

A waiting room with a children's play corner

6 Dealing with anxious patients

Dr Graham is talking about patient anxiety and how doctors deal with it nowadays.

A 22 Listen to what he says and match the improvements to how things were 30 years ago.

30 years ago	today
1 injections were painful	a doctors listen to patients more
2 doctors spent less time with patients	b smaller needles
3 doctors didn't explain things to patients	c surgeries have TVs and music
4 big, scary instruments	d smaller and less invasive instruments
5 not a relaxed atmosphere	e doctors should take more time to explain treatments

B Now write sentences with your answers. Start like this …

1 In the past, injections and taking blood were painful but now needles are smaller and cause less pain.
2 Today, doctors should spend more time talking to their patients.
3 …

7 Over to you

What are patients worried about nowadays when they visit the doctor? How can a doctor and/or medical assistant help anxious patients?

22 Listen to Dr Graham again and take notes. Then add your own ideas.

LANGUAGE

Nervous anxious patients need …		We could offer …
lots of	information	We should have …
	reassurance	… would be a good idea.
	…	… might help.

Modal verbs (Modalverben)

1 Doctors **should** always explain the risks and the benefits of each treatment.
2 The patients **have (got) to** trust you or they **shouldn't** start the treatment.
3 Some doctors still think they **don't have to** talk to their patients!
4 With today's anaesthetics, patients really **needn't** feel any pain at all.
5 Doctors **mustn't** forget to listen to their patients.

- *Should* drückt einen Ratschlag oder eine Empfehlung aus. (1)
- *Must* und *have (got) to* drücken eine Notwendigkeit bzw. Verpflichtung aus. (2)
- Die Verneinung von *must/have to* ist *don't have to* (3) bzw. *needn't* (4).
- Vorsicht: *mustn't* drückt ein Verbot aus (5) und bedeutet „nicht dürfen".

8 Practice

Choose the most suitable modal verb to complete the sentences.

1 With modern anaesthetics patients *needn't/mustn't* feel any pain.
2 Some doctors think they *don't have to/mustn't* listen to their patients.
3 Doctors *shouldn't/needn't* leave instruments lying around the surgery.
4 Patients *don't have to/must* go on with treatment if they feel nervous.
5 The sterilization centre *mustn't/needn't* be in the same room as the surgery.
6 Patients *don't have to/mustn't* have a reason for feeling anxious.
7 A doctor *needn't/shouldn't* look rushed or too busy.
8 People who are nervous about treatment *needn't/must* tell their doctor.

9 Situations

Work with a partner. Think of examples for the following things.

Something you …

1 shouldn't do at work.
2 don't have to do at home (but your partner does).
3 must do every day at work (but your partner doesn't).
4 have to do this weekend.

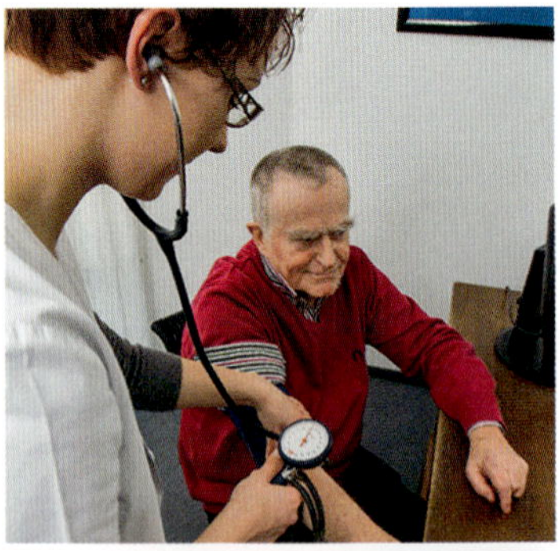

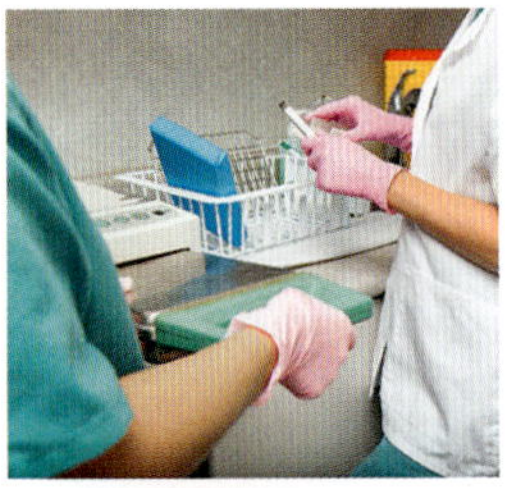

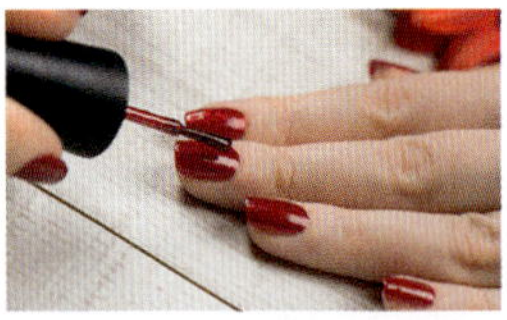

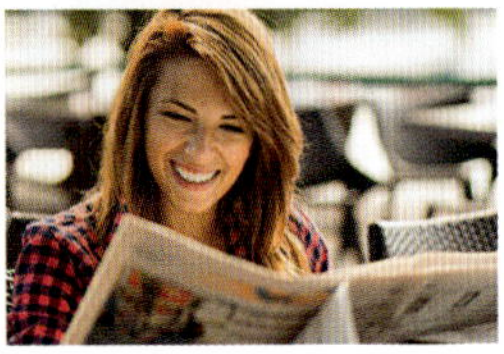

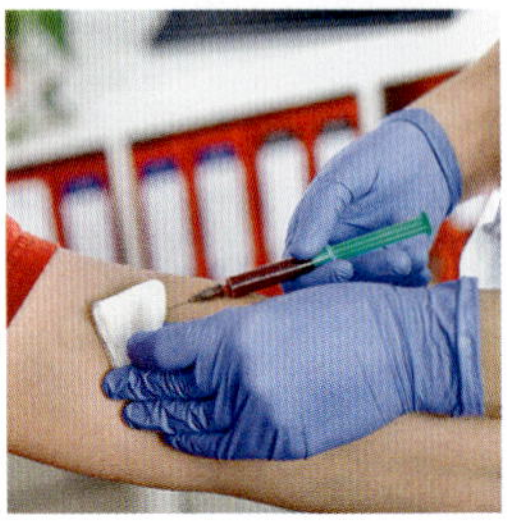

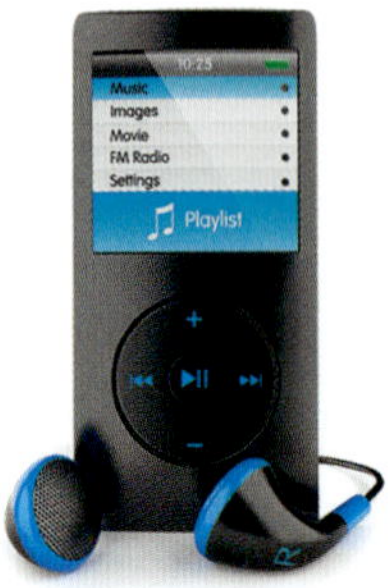

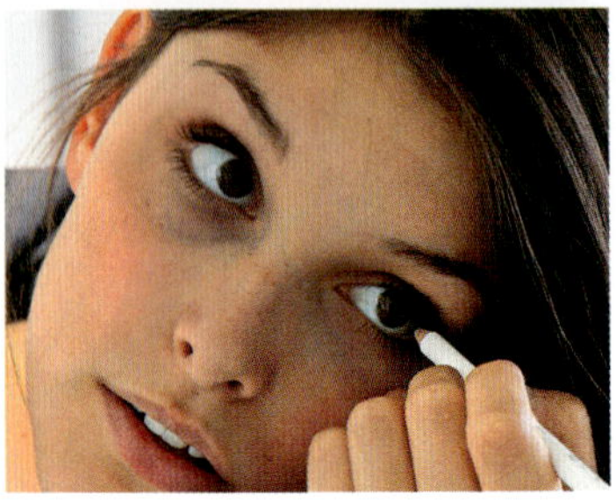

10 The pelvic examination

This is an examination that often causes anxiety and distress among women, and medical assistants need to calm and reassure patients.

Work with a partner. Discuss the following questions in German.

1 Why is it a good idea for young women to have a pelvic exam regularly?
2 When should a young woman go to the doctor for her first pelvic exam?

11 A first pelvic examination

Susan Farrows, 16, has arrived at the gynaecologist's surgery for her first pelvic examination. Meike, the medical assistant, talks to her.

23 Listen and take notes on what happens during the exam.

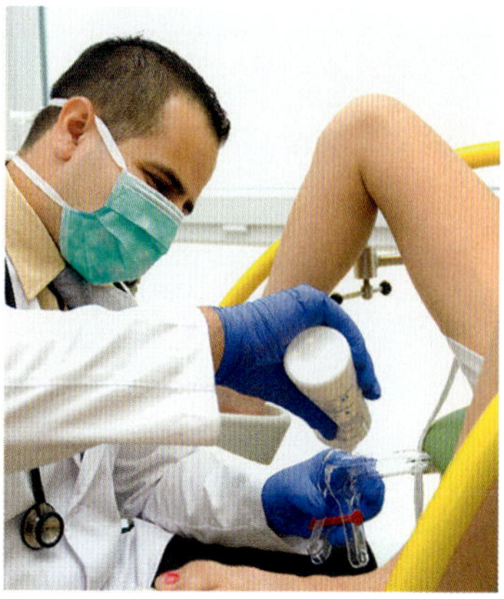

LANGUAGE

Reassuring patients
There's nothing to worry about. Don't worry, it's just a …
It's just a …, it won't hurt.
It's a very routine test / procedure / operation. It's perfectly normal.

12 Situations

Work with a partner. Pam, a fifteen-year-old Australian, comes for an HPV* test and vaccination.

Make up a dialogue between her and the medical assistant.

Medical assistant

Greet Pam and ask for name and appointment time.

Pam

Greet receptionist and give your name and the time of your appointment.

Medical assistant

Ask if it is her first visit to the surgery.

Pam

Say no, you have been before for a pelvic exam.

Medical assistant

Ask if the appointment is for another check-up.

Pam

Say no and explain that this time it is for an HPV* test and a vaccination. Add that you are a bit anxious.

Medical assistant

Reassure her by explaining the procedure.

* HPV = human papilloma virus. There are several different viruses and HPV16 and HPV18, are known to cause about 70% of cervical cancer. The use of the HPV test, also called Pap test, has led to a significant reduction in this form of cancer.

13 Dosage instructions

Sometimes when patients are anxious, they don't listen properly to what the doctor is saying. And if they listen, they often forget important information very quickly.

A Read the dialogue about a medical assistant giving dosage information to Pam, who is still a little anxious, and note down what she does to make sure that Pam remembers the instructions. Compare your notes with a partner.

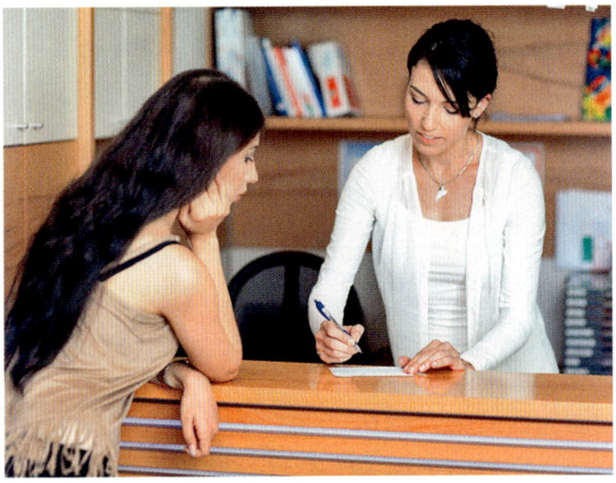

MFA So, Pam, here is your prescription. Please follow the dosage instructions very carefully.
Pam But I don't understand German very well.
MFA OK, no problem. So, let me explain. You have to take one tablet, three times a day. OK? And you have to take the tablet before eating and you take it with a some water. Do you understand?
Pam Yes.
MFA So that's one tablet, three times a day. Take it with water and before food. Here, let me write that down for you so you don't forget. And keep taking the tablets until they are all finished. Here you are.
Pam Thank you.
MFA The tablets might make you feel a little sleepy, but don't worry, that's normal. Do you have any questions about the tablets?
Pam No, I understand. Thank you.
MFA No problem. Have a good day, Pam.
Pam Thank you. Goodbye.

B An anxious patient, who speaks little German, comes back to the surgery having just collected his/her prescription from the local pharmacy.

Work with a partner to make a dialogue, as outlined on page 53. Use any parts of the dosage instructions there. The words and phrases in the box below will help you.

> ! prescription = Rezept
> recipe = (Koch-)Rezept

LANGUAGE

Taking medicine
Unless otherwise prescribed … Take with / before / after / meals.
Take once or twice a day.
Take a pill regularly every three hours. This capsule should be taken with some / lots of fluid / some water.

Do not take on an empty stomach / with other medication.
Dissolve in water. / Allow to dissolve in the mouth.
Swallow the tablet with water.

Side effects: in a minority of cases this medicine may cause …
drowsiness / nausea / stomach complaints / blurred vision / …

> ! You take something *for* a headache or *for* a pain in the back – not ~~against~~.

> ! You take medicine every three hours and not ~~all three hours~~.

1 **Dosierungsanleitung, Art und Dauer der Anwendung**
Soweit nichts anders verordnet, 3-5-mal täglich 20-30 Tropfen (1/2 Teelöffel) mit etwas Flüssigkeit oder auf Zucker vor den Mahlzeiten einnehmen. Die Anwendung erfolgt bis zur Beendigung der Beschwerden.

2 Eine Tablette einmal täglich während der Mahlzeit einnehmen. Nicht auf nüchternen Magen einnehmen, da Magenbeschwerden und Übelkeit auftreten können.

3 3–4-mal täglich 1 Kapsel eine halbe Stunde vor dem Essen mit reichlich kalter Flüssigkeit einnehmen. Zur Erleichterung der Nachtruhe kann die letzte Dosis vor dem Schlafengehen eingenommen werden.

4 **Nebenwirkungen**
In seltenen Fällen Magenbeschwerden und Übelkeit.

5 Erwachsene und Jugendliche ab 14 Jahren nehmen 2-3-mal täglich 1 Brausetablette ein. Kinder von 2-5 Jahren nehmen 3-mal täglich 1/2 Brausetablette oder 2-mal täglich 1 Brausetablette ein. Die Brausetabletten werden nach dem Mahlzeit in 1/2 Glas Wasser aufgelöst und die Lösung getrunken. Bei akuten Erkrankungen werden die Brausetabletten im Allgemeinen über 5-7 Tage eingenommen. Die Dauer der Behandlung richtet sich nach Art und Schwere der Erkrankung und sollte vom behandelnden Arzt bestimmt werden.

Medical assistant

Begrüßen Sie den Patienten / die Patientin.

Patient

Sagen Sie, Sie haben soeben Ihr Rezept von der Apotheke geholt aber haben eine Frage dazu.

Erkundigen Sie sich nach seiner/ihrer Frage.

Erklären Sie, dass Sie die Anweisungen nicht ganz verstehen, da Ihr Deutsch noch nicht gut genug ist.

Erklären Sie die Dosierung und wann das Medikament zu nehmen ist.

Fragen Sie nach der Dauer der Anwendungen.

Erklären Sie die Anwendung.

Fragen Sie nach Nebenwirkungen des Medikaments.

Beantworten Sie die Frage.

Sagen Sie, Sie haben es jetzt verstanden und drücken Sie Ihren Dank für die Hilfe aus.

Sagen Sie, dass dies Sie freut und verabschieden Sie sich.

Verabschieden Sie sich.

Exam Practice: A2 and B1

14 Leseverstehen: A2

Situation: Einer Ihrer Kollegen besuchte eine Fachtagung, auf der nur Englisch gesprochen wurde. Er hörte sich einen Vortrag zum Thema „Making Patients Feel Comfortable" an und machte sich dabei Notizen, die viele Ratschläge für Medizinische Fachangestellte beinhalten.

→ **Verwenden Sie diese Liste für einen kurzen Ratgeber für Berufsanfänger in deutscher Sprache:**

- Greet patients with a smile.
- Address them with their family name (surname).
- Reception room: Create a warm atmosphere (think about light, temperature, pictures, plants, magazines).
- Limit the amount of instruments and equipment that are within the sight of patients in the treatment or consultation room.
- Prepare patients for the check-up by telling them what to expect.
- Use words like "uncomfortable" rather than the more negative word "painful".
- Use physiological aids, if necessary (warmth, cold, etc.).
- Hold the hand of a nervous or very young patient during an injection or a vaccination and perhaps say something funny.
- Calm the patient by saying that everything will be fine.
- Stay with the patient or observe the patient until the medication or anaesthetics work.

15 Produktion: B1

Situation: Auf einer Urlaubsreise freundeten Sie sich mit Marsha aus London an, die genau wie Sie als Medizinische Fachangestellte tätig ist. Des Öfteren tauschen Sie in E-Mails Ihre beruflichen Erfahrungen aus. In Marshas letzter stellte Sie Ihnen die Frage, wie Sie mit ängstlichen Patienten umgehen.

→ **Antworten Sie Marsha per E-Mail und schildern darin aufgrund Ihrer bisherigen beruflicher Erfahrung, was Sie in einer dieser Situationen getan haben bzw. tun würden:**

- Ein 12-jähriger Junge kommt allein in Ihre Praxis. Er ist bei Glatteis ausgerutscht und hat Schmerzen im rechten Arm.
- Eine Schwangere ist beim Einkaufen im Supermarkt ohnmächtig geworden und wurde vom Marktleiter persönlich in Ihre Praxis gebracht.
- Eine ältere Dame kommt aufgeregt in Ihre Praxis, weil sie soeben von einem Hund gebissen wurde.

Führen Sie für die von Ihnen ausgewählte Situation drei Maßnahmen an.

16 The patient-carer relationship

A You are going to hear Joyce Reynolds give a presentation to people training to work in health and social care about the relationship between patients and carers.

Before listening, work with a partner to make a list of things that can go wrong in a patient-carer relationship. How do you think these problems can be avoided?

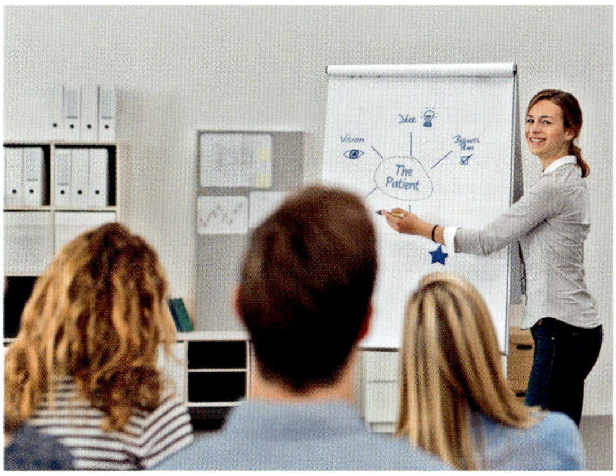

B 24 Now listen to the talk and put these headings into the correct order.

be honest • let clients do things for themselves • look after yourself • be patient and calm • take time to listen

C Try and complete the verb phrases below that you heard during the talk. Then listen again and check your answers.

1	rely	a	their self-respect
2	show	b	the truth
3	keep	c	warmth
4	don't reduce	d	care of yourself
5	put	e	calm
6	tell	f	sure
7	take	g	things right
8	make	h	on trust

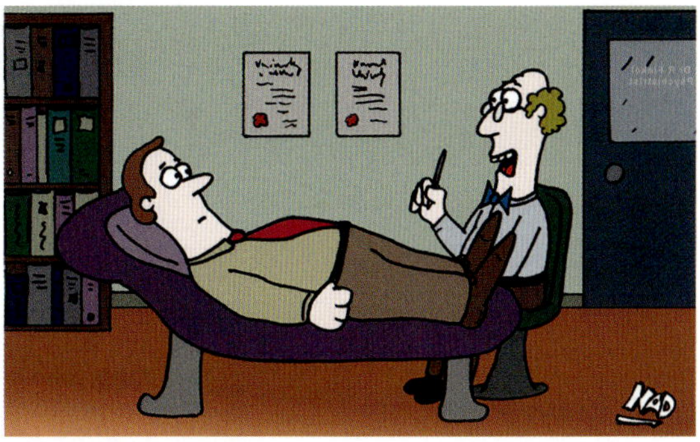

"Obsessive compulsive, anxious, paranoid and mildly psychotic ... but enough about me, let's talk about you!"

17 Preparing a presentation

You have been asked to give a short presentation to the class about the relationship between a medical assistant and patients at the practice.

Find information on the internet to help you and include the following in your presentation:

- why communication with patients is so important
- three key things to always remember when talking to patients
- where people can find out more information on this topic

7 Nutrition

1 Discussing a healthy diet

Scientific studies in the UK and the USA show that children who eat mainly junk food are more obese than children with healthier diets. At school their concentration is poorer and they are more badly behaved.

Work with a partner. Look at the quiz questions and decide which is the correct answer. Use the expressions in the Language box below.

1 How often should you eat fish?

a) once a week
b) twice a week
c) every day

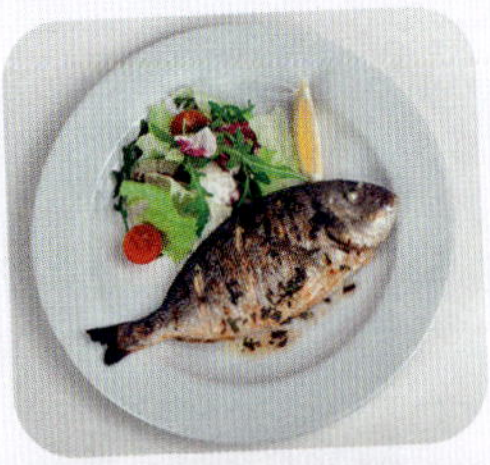

2 What contains the most vitamin C?

a) plums
b) oranges
c) kiwis

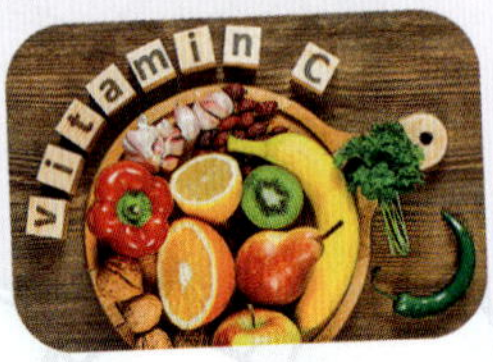

3 How much water should you drink every day?

a) 1 litre
b) 2 litres
c) 3 litres

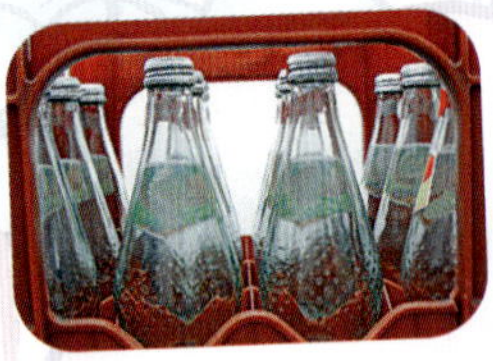

4 How much calcium does a body need to be healthy?

a) 250 mg a day
b) 500 mg a day
c) 1000 mg a day

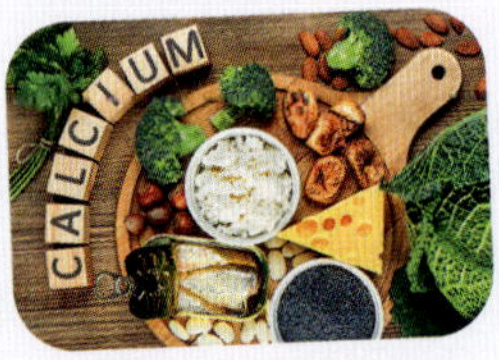

5 What percentage of our daily calorie intake (energy) should come from carbohydrates?

a) more than 50 per cent
b) more than 80 per cent
c) 100 per cent

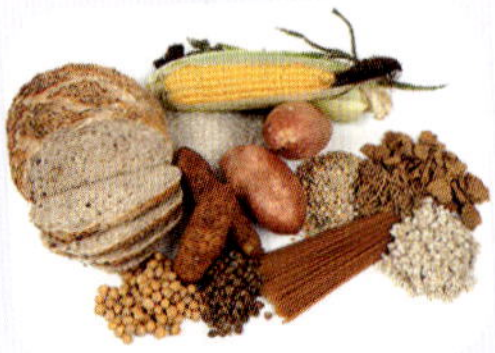

LANGUAGE

Agreeing and disagreeing
How do you feel about …?
I think that's right/wrong. What about you?
Do you agree?
I agree (with you).
I'm sorry, I don't agree. / I disagree.
I think …

2 A healthy diet

A Match the food items below to the six food groups in the healthy diet chart. Which food items can't be matched to the chart? Give reasons for your choice.

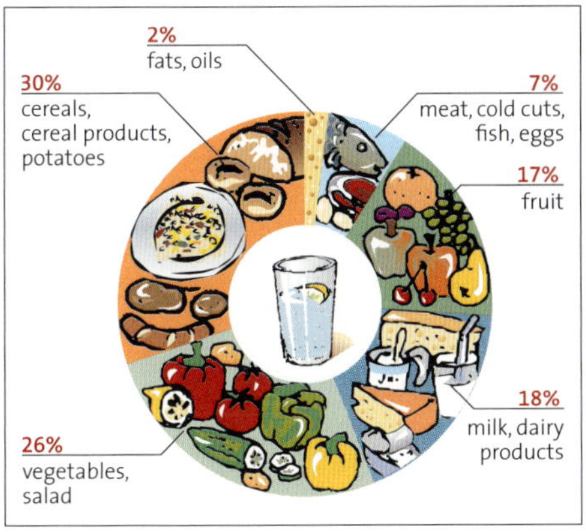

spaghetti • bananas • salt • cream • sugar • wine • cornflakes • chocolate • biscuits • bread rolls • orange juice • beer • salmon • chicken • broccoli • cola • sausage • onions • maple syrup

Complete this sentence:

Food items which contain ___, ___ or ___ should only be consumed in small amounts.

B Now add three items to each group. Use a dictionary to help you.

3 A nutrition hotline

Three people call the NHS Nutrition Hotline for advice about food.

A 25 Listen and match the items below to the telephone calls.

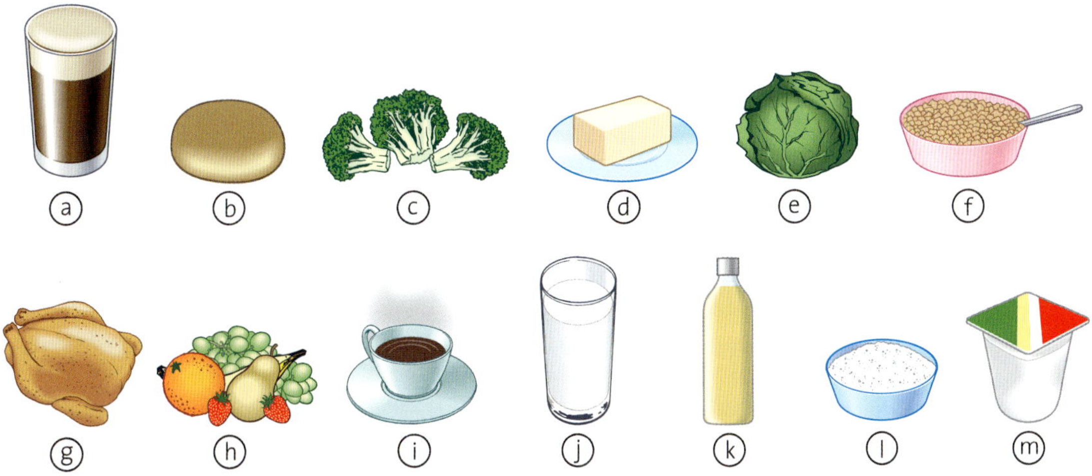

B Now listen to the three calls again and say whether the following statements are true or false. Correct the false statements.

1 High-fibre foods are some of the healthiest during pregnancy.
2 Vitamin D can be more harmful than vitamin A.
3 Coconut oil is healthier than olive oil.
4 Rapeseed oil and canola oil are the same.
5 Sweet teas are worse for your teeth than unsweetened teas.
6 Teas sweetened with sugar are some of the most popular baby products.

4 Working with words

Match the words with the definitions.

1	diet	a	to keep below a certain amount
2	cholesterol	b	to tell someone that something is good
3	fibre	c	breakfast food made from grains
4	to recommend	d	to make something higher
5	pregnancy	e	part of food that can also be found in the blood
6	to increase	f	what you eat
7	harmful	g	food or drink without sugar
8	to limit	h	when you are expecting a baby
9	cereals	i	bad for you
10	unsweetened	j	a harmful substance in the blood

Comparatives and superlatives (Steigerung der Adjektive)

1 Some fruit teas are **sweeter** than the unsweetened teas.
2 Let's all try and lead **healthier** lives.
3 Animal fat is **more harmful** than vegetable oil.
4 They are one of the **most popular** baby products.
5 Unsweetened teas are **better** for babies than sweet teas.

- Die meisten einsilbigen Adjektive und alle zweisilbigen Adjektive mit den Endungen *-y*, *-er* und *-ow* werden mit *-(e)r*, *-(e)st* gesteigert. (1, 2)
- Die meisten zweisilbigen und alle mehrsilbigen Adjektive werden mit *more/most*, *less/least* gesteigert. (3, 4)
- Ausnahmen sind *good – better – best; bad – worse – worst* und *little – less – least*. (5)
- *größer als* = bigger than, not ~~bigger as~~

5 Practice

Complete the sentences using a comparative or superlative form.

1 Skimmed milk is ___ (healthy) than full fat milk.
2 Saturated fats are the ___ (dangerous) type of fats.
3 People with heart disease often have ___ (high) cholesterol levels than normal.
4 Vitamin C and D are ___ (good) for you than vitamin B.
5 Some fruit teas have ___ (little) sugar in them than other sweetened teas.
6 Heart disease is one of the ___ (big) killers in Europe.
7 Eating the right food is ___ (important) than how much you eat.
8 Baby food in a jar is ___ (quick) to prepare than fresh food.
9 A diet rich in folic acid is ___ (good) for pregnant women.
10 Saturated fats are ___ (harmful) than vegetable oils.
11 Bread and cereals are ___ (high) in fibre than fruit.
12 Smoking is one of the ___ (bad) things for a pregnant woman.
13 Is honey more or ___ (harmful) for babies than sugar?
14 A-Z medical insurance offers you the ___ (good) treatment for the ___ (little) cost.
15 Mr Castle's condition hasn't improved and is now ___ (bad) than before.

6 Talking about diabetes

In the UK there are over 2.5m people diagnosed with diabetes and a further half a million who have the disease but don't know it.

A Work with a partner. Produce a list of all the words in the text that have something to do with illness.

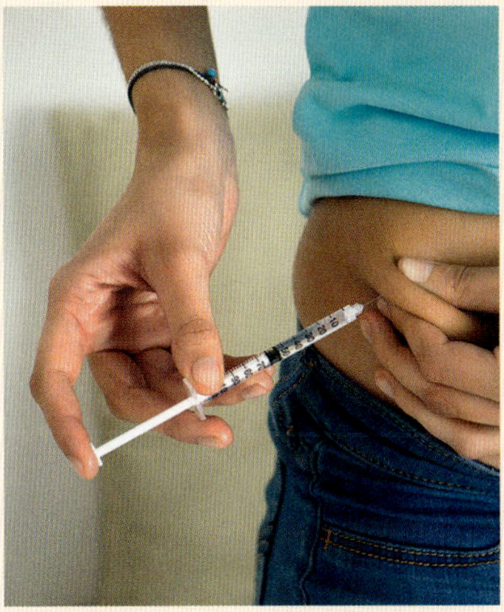

The truth about diabetes

With so much information about diabetes out there, be sure you're getting the correct facts. Here are some answers to some commonly asked questions.

Although we don't know why some people get diabetes, we know it is not contagious – it can't be caught like a cold or the flu.
Diabetes is caused by a combination of genetic and environmental factors. However, a diet high in fat and sugar can cause you to become overweight. Being overweight increases your risk of developing Type 2 diabetes.

There is no such thing as a mild form of diabetes. All diabetes is equally serious, and if not properly controlled can lead to serious health problems.
If you have good control of your diabetes, you will be able to live a completely normal and full life. Research shows, for example, that people with diabetes are no less safe on the roads than anyone else. However, in the UK, people who treat their diabetes with insulin injections are not allowed to drive buses or coaches.

Diabetes, when properly controlled, should also not stop people from taking part in exercise or sport. Ask Steve Redgrave, the five-times Olympic gold medal-winning rower; or many of the other people with diabetes who take part in the London Marathon every year. People with diabetes should do exercise as part of a healthy lifestyle.

You are not more likely to get a cold or another illness if you have diabetes. But people with diabetes are advised to get flu jabs. This is because any infection changes their blood glucose-control, putting them at risk of high blood glucose levels.

Sweets and other sugary foods are no more dangerous for people with diabetes than they are for the rest of us, if they're part of a healthy diet. Remember that confectionery foods are also higher in fat and calories, and this is the reason why you shouldn't eat too many, especially if you are trying to lose weight.

B Do you know the opposite of these words? If you need help, you will find them in the text on page 59.

1 incorrect
2 low
3 underweight
4 decrease
5 dangerous
6 unhealthy

Diabetes facts

- In 2015 an estimated 415m people had diabetes worldwide.
- This is equal to 8.3% of the world's adult population.
- This is estimated to rise to 592m people by 2035.
- Type 2 diabetes accounts for 90% of cases.
- As many men have diabetes as women.
- Diabetes is estimated to result in 2-5m deaths a year.
- The global economic cost of diabetes is $612bn a year.

7 Odd one out

A **Find the word that doesn't fit. Give a reason for your choice.**

1	a lead to	b catch	c cause
2	a cold	b diabetes	c flu
3	a environmental	b controlled	c safe
4	a diet	b sport	c exercise
5	a genetic	b contagious	c infectious
6	a risk	b danger	c health
7	a sugar	b fibre	c glucose
8	a lifestyle	b jab	c injection
9	a sweets	b chocolates	c calories
10	a fruit	b glucose	c sugar

B **Complete the sentences with words from exercise A.**

1 A ___ high in fat and sugar can make you overweight.
2 A good diet and exercise are part of a healthy ___.
3 Diabetes is not ___ – you can't get it from other people like a cold.
4 If someone with diabetes gets the flu, it can cause high blood ___ levels.
5 All forms of diabetes can ___ serious health problems if not controlled.
6 People can be very active and still do ___ if they have diabetes.
7 Catching ___ can cause problems with blood glucose control.
8 Eating ___ every day is good for you, but please remember it also contains sugar.
9 For some people, their diabetes must be ___ by insulin injections.
10 Three pieces of chocolate contain over 50 ___.

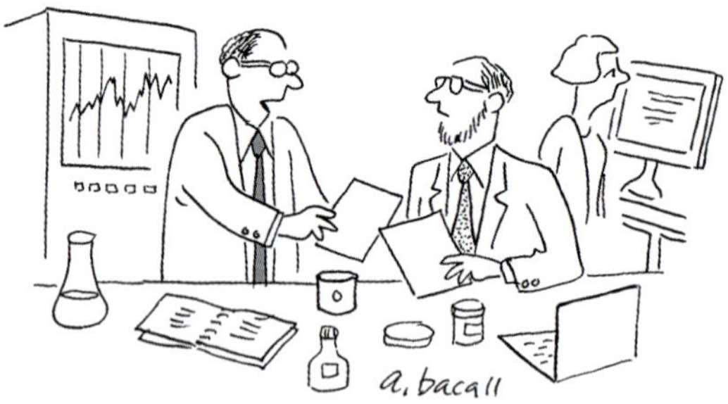

"My diabetic research shows that test subjects are 98% more likely to take their diabetic pills if the pills are covered in chocolate."

8 Controlling diabetes

Magda Jakimowicz is a Polish national living in Germany. She has just been diagnosed with Type 2 diabetes and is talking to a medical assistant about how to control her condition.

26))) Listen to or read the dialogue and answer the questions below.

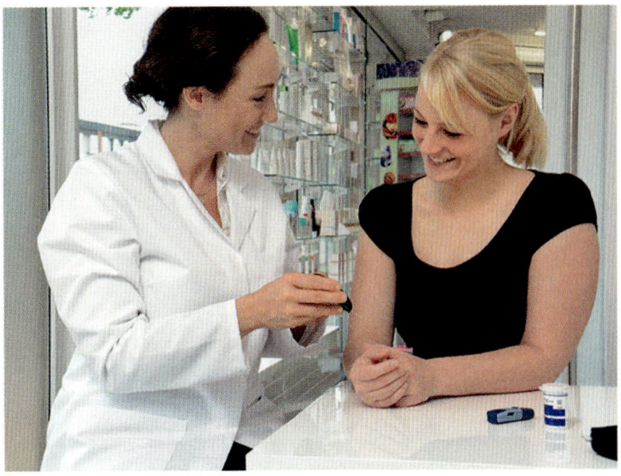

Assistant So, you've seen the doctor. Was it all OK?

Magda Yes, he told me to speak to you about things I can do every day to help.

Assistant Did he say if you need tablets or insulin injections?

Magda He's prescribed some tablets, but I don't need injections.

Assistant That's good news. One of the most important things is to take day-to-day control of your diabetes yourself and make the right changes to your lifestyle.

Magda Do you mean don't eat chocolate and things like that?

Assistant No, chocolate is actually OK – but just make sure you limit it to small amounts. What you need to do is to pay attention to things like a healthy diet, losing a bit of weight and more physical activity.

Magda Is that all?

Assistant That and learning about self-care. I'll give you some information on diet and how you can learn to monitor your own blood glucose levels. There are some really simple things you can do like checking your feet for signs of high blood glucose levels.

Magda My feet?

Assistant I know! It sounds crazy but it's true. It's all in the information here. You'll need to work with your diabetes care team – that's us. Talk regularly with us and learn when to ask for help if you're ill or get a chest infection, for example. We'll make some regular appointments and it's really important that you keep them so that the team knows you're making the right changes to your daily lifestyle and your diabetes is under control. Type 2 diabetes is progressive – so if you don't control it, it can get worse and cause damage to your nerves, heart and arteries.

1 What medicine did the doctor prescribe Magda?
2 Magda needs to make simple changes to her daily lifestyle. What are they?
3 What kind of self-care information do you think the assistant gives Magda?
4 When does Magda need to speak to her care team?
5 Explain what is meant by 'Type 2 diabetes is progressive'.

9 Self-care information

Use the information in the dialogue to create a self-care information leaflet for a Type 2 diabetes patient. Think about:

- the changes they need to make themselves
- the support they will get
- when to ask for help
- why it's important to follow the advice

10 Mediation: A2

Situation: Mit Ihren Praktikantinnen aus Malaysia und Polen verbringen Sie die Mittagspause meist im Schnellrestaurant. Demnächst eröffnet nebenan ein Restaurant mit dem „Slow Food"-Konzept. Ihre Kolleginnen und Kollegen meinen, dass die Mittagspause auf mehrere Stunden ausgedehnt werden müsste, wenn man dort Gast sein wollte. Sie wissen es jedoch besser, weil Sie den untenstehenden Text gelesen haben.

→ **Erstellen Sie Präsentationsfolien in englischer Sprache für eine Mitarbeiterbesprechung anhand des deutschen Textes über „Slow Food".**

Slow Food steht für genussvolles, bewusstes und regionales Essen und bezeichnet eine Gegenbewegung zum weltweit gleichen Fastfood. Es kommen nur Zutaten aus der näheren Umgebung in Frage – und auch nur solche, die zur betreffenden Jahreszeit vorrätig sind. Die Zubereitungsmethode ist vorwiegend traditionell. Die ursprünglich aus Italien stammende Bewegung bemüht sich um die Erhaltung der regionalen Küche mit heimischen pflanzlichen und tierischen Produkten und deren lokale Produktion, also gut, sauber und fair. Wenn eines dieser Elemente fehlt, handelt es sich nicht um Slow Food.

11 Produktion: B1

Situation: Einer Ihrer Freunde wird demnächst ein kleines Restaurant eröffnen. Er hat sich entschieden, das Konzept „Slow Food" umzusetzen. Die Gerichte sollen preiswert und schmackhaft sein. Zudem sollen die Zutaten nur von Händlern mit dem Gütesiegel „Fair Trade" bezogen werden.
Das Restaurant soll am 15. des nächsten Monats eröffnet werden. Es soll ein Flyer gedruckt werden, der an alle Haushalte in der näheren Umgebung verteilt wird – und zwar sowohl in deutscher als auch englischer Sprache. Für den englischen Text hat er sich den Slogan:

IN A HURRY? THEN PLEASE DO NOT BE OUR GUEST!

ausgedacht. Für den dazugehörigen Text bittet er Sie um Hilfe.

→ **Schreiben Sie den gewünschten Text, in dem Sie das Konzept „Slow Food" erläutern und alle Informationen der obigen Situationsbeschreibung verwenden.**

Did TV chef lose the fight for healthier school dinners?

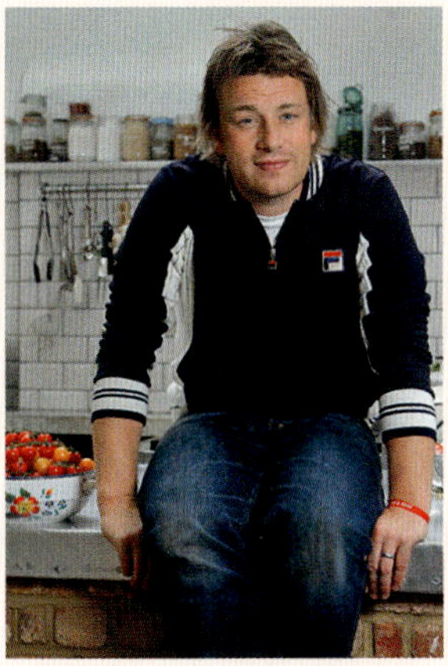

In 2005, TV chef Jamie Oliver, led a high-profile TV campaign to introduce healthier eating habits into schools in England. Oliver started his **Feed Me Better** campaign because of the junk food being served in many English schools. His hit television programme **Jamie's School Dinners** saw him asking children to eat salads and fruit rather than chips and burgers. Schools also looked at banning crisps, confectionery and snacks as well as sugary and carbonated drinks.

The award-winning television show, which had millions of viewers, reported that the average school dinner was very low-cost, and this led to the government to provide a multi-million financial injection to improve school dinners in England. The show also led to the introduction of healthy school dinner guidelines that banned certain junk foods and sugary drinks. In 2009, a report showed a 6% improvement in maths and English exam results in those schools that followed the new guidelines.

But despite these victories and the popularity of the TV show, a report in 2009 showed a 17% drop in the number of children eating school dinners since the healthy guidelines were introduced. The report spoke of a growing black market for non-nutritional foods, problems with burger vans outside schools, and chips being passed through school gates. Schools also lost up to £12,000 a year by not being able to sell junk food and fizzy drinks.

A change of government saw an end to the extra funding of school dinners in 2009. The following year the government also decided not to apply the healthy guidelines to many schools in England. In 2015 Jamie Oliver himself said he thought the campaign had failed. In a radio interview, Oliver said: "In Britain, eating well and feeding your kid right and being aware about food is all considered very posh and middle class, but the reality is that in most of Europe some of the best food comes from the poorest communities." He has now recently embarked on a new project to rid children's diets of excess sugar, as he argues its effect on public health today is "extraordinary".

12 Working with words

Read the article and match the words and phrases (1–6) with the definitions (a–f).

1 to ban	**a** to say something must not be done
2 guidelines	**b** a drink with small bubbles
3 victory	**c** instructions about the best way to do something
4 black market	**d** to begin something
5 fizzy	**e** success when you win something
6 to embark on	**f** place where you can illegally buy things that are hard to get

13 A discussion of the pros and cons

Work with a partner. First make notes, then discuss whether the campaign has been a success or not.

8 Eating disorders

1 Symptoms of eating disorders

You hear a radio interview at work with a health expert talking about eating disorders.

A 27 Listen and match the symptoms to the disorders. Some symptoms are in more than one category.

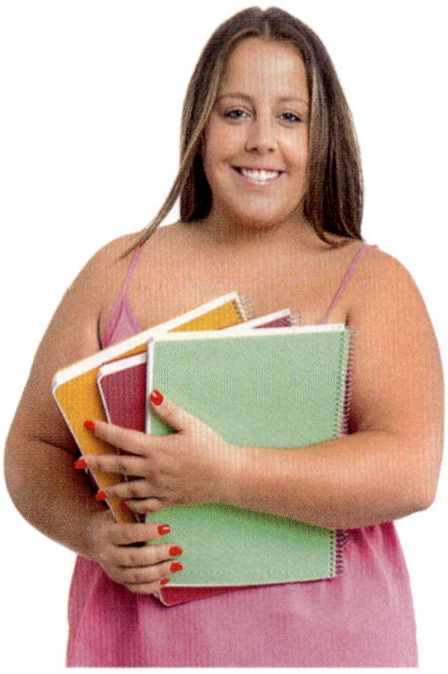

Eating disorders:

anorexia nervosa	bulimia	overeating

Symptoms:

- a depression
- b fast or irregular heart rate
- c dental problems
- d low blood pressure
- e poor circulation
- f purging / controlled vomiting
- g frequent headaches
- h hair loss
- i hair growth on face
- j no energy or enthusiasm
- k feeling cold
- l high blood pressure

B Work with a partner and answer the following questions.

1 Why is the number of people with an eating disorder growing?
2 What is 'purging'?
3 Why do you think parents 'often don't see the symptoms'?
4 Why do bulimics eat 'large amounts of food'?
5 What problems can obesity cause?
6 What should parents do if they notice symptoms of an eating disorder?

Eating disorders

- Obesity kills 35,000 people a year in the UK.
- You are obese if you have a Body Mass Index (weight in kilograms divided by the square of your height in metres) of 30 or more.
- About 165,000 people in the UK suffer from eating disorders. 1 in 10 are men.
- Eating disorders kill around 19,000 people a year in the UK.

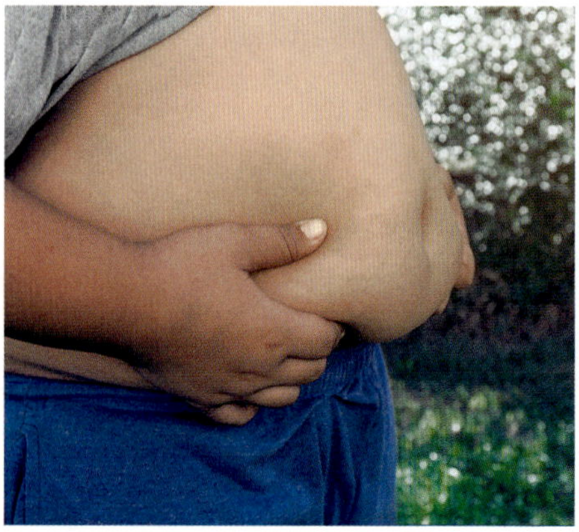

2 Dealing with eating disorders

A Read the text below and match the headings (a–e) to the paragraphs 1–5.

- **a** Provide a healthy family environment
- **b** Be sensitive to their emotions
- **c** Ask for professional help
- **d** Encourage their creative abilities
- **e** Don't ignore the signs

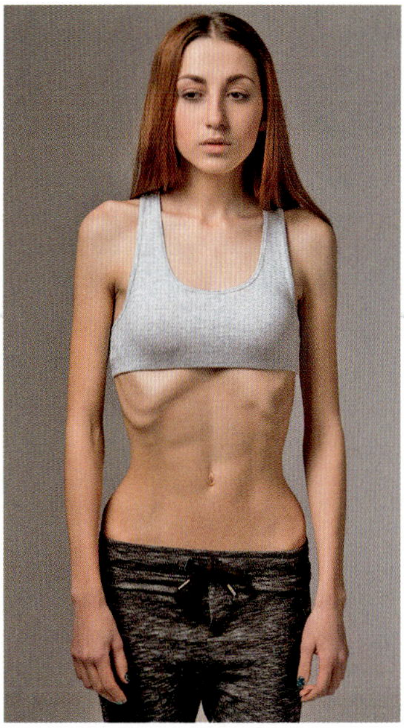

Teenage Eating Disorders – What can the family do? Statistics show that about 10% of the U.S. population suffers from some form of eating disorder. Almost 95% of sufferers are women, most of them aged between 10 and 20. For families who have teenagers suffering from these disorders, here are the steps that can be taken to address the problem before it gets worse.

1 Treatment clinics for people suffering from eating problems can be found everywhere. These facilities generally offer psychological counselling, nutritional therapy and medical attention.

2 If you think that your adolescent child is just picky with his or her food, you might miss the chance to treat the disorder when it starts, which is always the best time to deal with the problem. Look for symptoms, like being too worried about body weight, obsession with counting calories and weighing food, uncontrolled eating or dieting, vomiting or purging and extreme mood swings.

3 Eating disorders can start because of a traumatic experience. Experts say that some people who suffer from one of these disorders have been abused as a child. Teenage girls and boys who have experienced failure and humiliation also sometimes turn to overeating or not eating at all as a way of dealing with their emotions.

4 Don't try to avoid family problems. If there are big changes within the family that can hurt your teenager, talk about them in the open and try to get them to talk about their feelings and say what they think about the situation. However, don't be too pushy as this is something that teenagers really don't like.

5 Letting teenagers do activities that they like and they are good at can give them a good emotional and psychological foundation. Encourage them to express their thoughts and ideas and do their hobbies, but don't make them live up to your personal expectations of them. Teenage eating disorders are not just physical health problems, they are primarily psychological and should be addressed by giving young people all the love and support that they need.

B Complete the table with the correct form of the words from the text on page 65.

verb	noun
populate	1 ___
counsel	2 ___
3 ___	treatment
obsess	4 ___
5 ___	abuse
fail	6 ___
7 ___	expression
expect	8 ___

C Working with words

Now use the words from B to complete the sentences.

1 The best time to ___ an eating disorder is when it first starts.
2 Experiencing humiliation or ___ can also lead to an eating disorder.
3 One symptom of a disorder is when someone shows an ___ with counting calories.
4 Some teenagers feel they can't live up to their parents' high ___ .
5 Many disorders are emotional and can be treated by psychological ___ .
6 People with eating problems often feel unable to ___ their thoughts and feelings.
7 Eating disorders are sometimes a result of child ___ .
8 Research shows that one tenth of the ___ in the USA has some form of eating disorder.

3 Discussing weight problems

The rate of childhood obesity in the USA tripled between 1980–2000 and today has reached 32%. In Germany the rate is 15% but growing. Your boss asks you to find out about the problem in the USA.

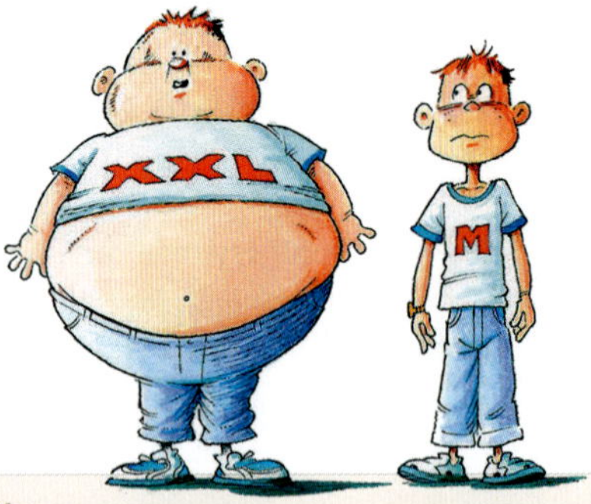

A 28 Listen to an expert from the US National Obesity Forum and complete the following sentences.

1 Kids in the USA are becoming ___ .
2 People are obese when their ___ is 30 or more.
3 Kids today do far less physical ___ .
4 They also eat less ___ food.
5 Kids copy each other's eating ___ .
6 Obesity increases the risk of type 2 ___ .
7 More than ___ Americans have diabetes.

B Listen again and say what the following numbers refer to in the dialogue.

a 10–17
b 49
c 30
d 18–25
e 37%
f 150bn

Global obesity

- Worldwide, approximately 1.9 billion adults are overweight.
- Worldwide obesity doubled in the years 1980–2014.
- 39% of adults are overweight. 13% are obese.
- 65% of the world's population lives in a country where obesity and being overweight kill more people than being underweight.

4 Psychological problems

You find an article in a medical journal about how to help someone with an eating disorder. The article lists the things you shouldn't say to someone with an eating disorder.

Work with a partner. Why shouldn't you say any of the things below to someone with an eating disorder? Read the article below and match 1–7 to the psychological problems (a–d).

1 Why are you doing this to me?
2 Are you sick?
3 I don't understand how you can eat so much.
4 You look like you've got AIDS.
5 If you love your family, eat something.
6 You'll make yourself sick if you don't eat.
7 That's why you haven't got many friends.

EATING DISORDERS AND THE MIND

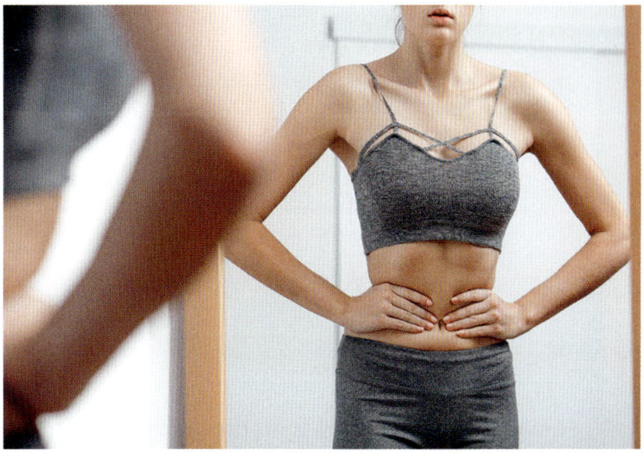

People who suffer from eating disorders DO NOT need to look underweight or act differently. Many men and women have normal body weight but can still suffer badly from any of these psychological problems.

a) Negative self-image
This includes feelings such as 'I never do anything right' or 'people will like me more if I lose weight'. Anorexics and bulimics often want everything to be perfect and they starve themselves or binge if they don't do things well. Overeaters are often called 'fat' or 'lazy', which makes them feel very lonely.

b) Guilt
People with eating disorders often worry about all of the problems they give their friends and family. They feel bad about not being a 'strong and normal person' and find it hard to meet the expectations of parents and friends.

c) Power
Anorexics and bulimics often experience highs after a binge. They think they are still in control of the problem if they can carefully plan their binges and purges. This feeling of control is all they have, and they fight people who try to take it away from them.

d) Depression
This includes low motivation, feelings of hopelessness, worrying about everything and feeling completely alone. In some cases, depression can even lead to people with eating disorders taking their own lives.

5 Working with words

Choose the correct word to complete the sentences.

1 Anorexics don't always look badly underweight/overweight.
2 Many eating disorders are caused by psychological/mind problems.
3 Anorexics can binge/starve themselves if things don't go well.
4 Overweight people are often called lonely/lazy.
5 Bulimics often feel guilty/alone about the problems they cause.

> **Calories**
>
> A calorie is a unit of energy. In nutrition and everyday language, calories refer to energy consumption through eating and drinking, and energy usage through physical activity. For example, an apple may have 80 calories (kcal), while a one-mile walk might use up about 100 calories (kcal).
>
> **A food calorie or kilogram calorie** (kcal) is the amount of energy required to raise the temperature of one kilogram of water by one degree Celsius.

> ***If*-clauses type 1 (*If*-Sätze)**
>
> 1 If I **lose** weight, people **will like** me more.
> 2 Sufferers **can die** if they don't respond to treatment.
> 3 They **are** still in control if they can carefully plan their binges.
> 4 If you love your family, **eat** something.
>
> – *If-clauses* vom Typ 1: *If*-Satz mit *simple present* – Hauptsatz mit *will* + Verb. (1)
> – Im Hauptsatz können anstelle von *will* andere Modalverben wie *can* (2), eine Gegenwartsform von *be* (3) und Verben in der Befehlsform (4) stehen.

6 Practice

Complete the following sentences with the correct form of the verbs.

1 If you ___ (be) worried about someone's eating, ___ (speak) to a doctor.
2 If sufferers ___ (take) their eating disorders seriously, they ___ (get) better.
3 Children ___ (be) more likely to be obese if they ___ (have) overweight friends.
4 Teenagers ___ (not/like) it if parents ___ (be) too pushy.
5 If you ___ (not/notice) the symptoms early, the problem ___ (get) worse.
6 If there ___ (be) changes in the family, ___ (talk) about them with your child.
7 Sometimes teenagers ___ (feel) guilty if they ___ (cause) problems at home.
8 Unfortunately, sometimes anorexics ___ (starve) themselves if things ___ (not/go) well.
9 ___ (talk) to your parents if you ___ (think) you have problems with food.

7 Internet research

In pairs, try and match the foods (1–8) with the number of calories per 100 grams (a–h). Check your answers by researching on the internet.

1 butter	5 skimmed milk	a 28	e 200
2 fried egg	6 chocolate biscuit	b 35	f 490
3 boiled egg	7 peanut butter	c 66	g 600
4 whole milk	8 apricot	d 160	h 770

8 Mediation

Situation: Sie haben seit vielen Jahren eine Brieffreundin Sheila in Manchester. Diese schrieb Ihnen vor einigen Monaten, dass sie sich ihrer Gesundheit zuliebe nur noch vegan ernähren wollte. Kürzlich schrieb sie jedoch, dass sie sich nicht besonders gut fühle und wandte sich mit der Bitte um einen Rat an Sie, weil Sie ja im Gesundheitsbereich arbeiten. Zufällig fanden Sie den unten stehenden Artikel in einer Tageszeitung und können sich vorstellen, dass Ihre Freundin zu viel des Guten getan hat.

→ Schreiben Sie Ihrer Brieffreundin eine E-Mail, in der Sie die Inhalte des deutschen Textes über Orthorexie (englisch: „Orthorexia") wiedergeben und geben ihr einen individuellen Rat, was sie Ihrer Meinung nach tun sollte. Übersetzen Sie den Text nicht, sondern verwenden Sie nur die darin enthaltenen Informationen für Ihre E-Mail!

Orthorexie

„Orthorexie ist eine Fixierung auf den Verzehr von ausschließlich gesunden Lebensmitteln", erklärt Friederike Barthels vom Institut für experimentelle Psychologie der Universität Düsseldorf. Dabei gibt es allerdings ein Problem: „Die Definition, was gesund ist, ist individuell verschieden. Dadurch besteht die Gefahr, dass es eben nicht mehr gesund ist, sondern sehr einseitig und sehr extrem."

„Betroffene verlieren oft die sozialen Kontakte, weil ein Restaurantbesuch mit Freunden und Familie für sie kaum noch möglich ist", erklärt Helmut Schatz, früherer Mediensprecher der Deutschen Gesellschaft für Endokrinologie, die sich mit Hormonen und dem Stoffwechsel beschäftigt. Orthorexie ist dem Experten zufolge zunächst einmal eine Essbesonderheit. „Stellt sich aber ein Zwang ein und leidet der Mensch darunter, dann wird es krankhaft."

9 Super slim me

A After the introduction, the following paragraphs in the article are mixed up. Read each one carefully and then put them in the correct order.

Super slim me

Despite young women starving themselves to death, the catwalks at London Fashion Week are still full of size zero models. TV presenter Dawn Porter finds out what life on a 'zero diet' is really like.

a 'But then a terrible thing started to happen. As the weight fell off me, I really liked how I looked. For the first time, my tummy was flat. Even though I was always hungry, I was excited to see how much more I could lose. I cut back to 400 calories a day – even going as low as 250 calories on some days. Suddenly I understood the madness of pro-anorexia websites and the results of starvation.'

b At the start of the challenge, Dawn weighed 63 kg with a BMI of 22 – which was the perfect weight for her height. 'When I took on the challenge of a starvation diet, I thought that hunger would be my biggest problem. The hunger actually became a sick comfort to me as the hungrier I was, the more I felt I was doing the right thing. I was on 500 calories a day and obsessing about what I was eating. I soon started to feel tired all the time as I couldn't sleep at night because of the permanent hunger.'

c 'Then my doctor advised me to stop. My mineral levels were dangerously low and I risked my periods stopping and my hair growing thin. I was suffering headaches and terrible constipation and my immune system was so weak I risked infection. My BMI was down to 18 and my dress size a UK 8, but my life was no better, or more successful than before. I'd never felt so unattractive and it was the worst time of my life.'

d In August 2006, 22-year-old Uruguayan model Luisel Ramos died after starving herself. She had tried to live on nothing but cola and lettuce leaves for three months. At the time of her death she had a BMI of 14.5. The World Health Organization considers a BMI of below 16 to be starvation. Six months later, her sister Eliana Ramos, 18, was found dead in her bedroom. She, too, had worked as a model and died of malnutrition and anorexia.

e 'But for all my joy of losing weight, by week seven the depression kicked in. I'd never suffered depression in my life, but suddenly I would cry for no reason. Even though I'd never looked so slim, I was more insecure about my body than ever before. I felt unattractive. I went out on a date, but it was a disaster because I talked about dieting and calories all night. Men didn't find me attractive and women were jealous of my thinness.'

f In order to find out exactly what young models such as the Ramos sisters must go through to become a size zero, TV presenter Dawn Porter went on a crash diet. For two months a film crew recorded her as she tried to go from a curvy UK size 12 to a super skinny size 4 (US size zero). 'My aim was to show what kind of a miserable life you have to lead, what food you must eat – or must not eat – and the exercise you must do if you want to be a size zero.'

B **Match the summaries (1–6) to the paragraphs (a–f).**

1 The effects of hunger
2 Why I had to stop the diet
3 Two models starve to death
4 My dieting success excited me
5 Depression kicks in
6 My crash diet and its aims

Dreams and reality

- 6% of women are underweight, but 44% are overweight.
- Around 40% of models have an eating disorder.
- The average American model is thinner than 98% of American women.
- Madrid Fashion Week only accepts models with a minimum BMI of 18.
- Vogue International does not feature models who are unnaturally thin.

C **Choose the correct words from the list to complete each sentence.**

anorexia · challenge · hungry · insecure · jealous · kicked in · low · permanent · skinny · starvation · tired · unattractive

1 When talking with friends, I was always obesssing about food and trying not to eat, but I was so ___.
2 When I reached size 8, friends started to say I looked so thin and ___.
3 I was constantly hungry and couldn't sleep because of the ___ hunger.
4 At less than 500 calories a day I was on a ___ diet.
5 After a few weeks the depression ___ and I felt really down.
6 I obsessed about food and was unhappy and ___ about how I looked.
7 Many women are ___ of other women who are slim.
8 Despite losing weight I didn't feel I looked good, in fact I felt the exact opposite: ___ .
9 I thought the biggest ___ would be the hunger.
10 I felt ___ all the time because I couldn't sleep.
11 Malnutrition and ___ are two problems we have to take very seriously.
12 The World Health Organization says a BMI below 16 is dangerously ___.

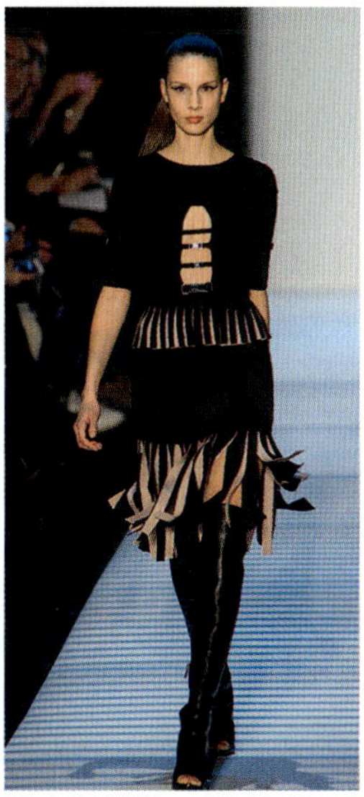

10 Producing a webpage: Eating disorders

Your practice is near an international school and your boss has asked you to produce a webpage in English with the title 'What parents should know about eating disorders'.

Look at all the information in the unit and include the following:

- tips on how to recognize eating disorders
- advice on how to deal with them
- links to some national and international organizations that help sufferers
- advice and support for their families

9 Screening for illness

1 Screening for breast cancer

Shelly Brady is an American who is working in Freiburg. She goes to see her gynaecologist, Dr Schneider.

A 29 Listen and write down the reason for Shelly's visit.

B What action is Dr Schneider going to take?

C Match the words that you heard in the recording with the definitions below.

1 lump
2 self-examination
3 fuss
4 suspicious
5 pressure
6 (medical) history
7 mammogram
8 (menstrual) cycle

a force or weight put on something
b an X-ray of the breast
c anxious behaviour about something that is unimportant
d monthly process of ovulation and menstruation in a woman's body
e giving you the feeling that something bad is happening
f when a woman checks her own breasts for any signs of cancer
g small piece of something solid, without a specific shape
h all the things that have happened in the past with someone's health

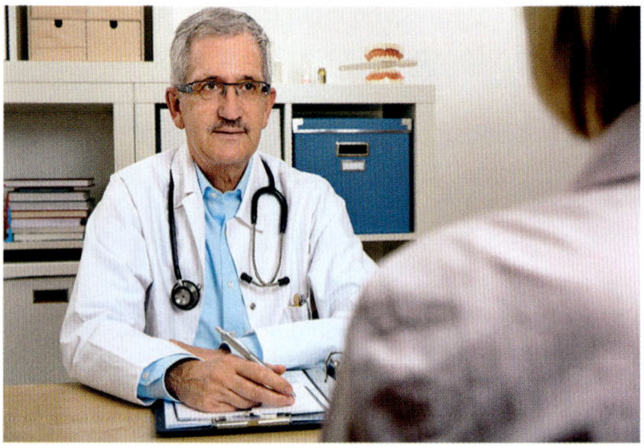

Breast screening UK

- 1 in 8 women are diagnosed with breast cancer in the UK.
- All women between 50–70 years old are automatically invited for a mammogram every two years.
- These are done in specialist clinics or mobile breast screening units.
- Results are always sent to the patient's GP within two weeks.

Breast screening USA

- 1 in 8 women are diagnosed with breast cancer in the USA.
- The American Cancer Society (ACS) recommends all women 45–74 years old have a mammogram every two years.
- These are done at mobile units, private radiology offices, hospital clinics or a doctor's office.
- Results are given immediately at the centre or sent to the patient's Primary Care Physician.

2 A breast examination

Dr Schneider is going to examine Shelly Brady.

30))) Listen (or read) and write down the steps that Dr Schneider follows when doing the examination.

Dr Schneider So, Mrs Brady, I'm going to examine your breasts to see if there is anything there for us to worry about. Is it OK for me to do this now or would you like someone else to be here, too?

Shelly Brady No, that's fine, Doctor. I'm OK with it.

Dr Schneider Right, good. If you'd like to just step into this treatment area here and please remove all your upper clothing, including your bra. I'm going to put this screen across to give you a little bit of privacy. There you are. I'll give you a minute to get undressed and then come and examine you. You can put your clothes on the chair there.

Shelly Brady OK, thanks.

Dr Schneider Right, let's take a look. I'm just going to feel in your armpits to begin with. If you could just raise your arm for me. That's it, thank you. I'm going to apply some gentle pressure here. Don't worry, it isn't going to hurt. OK, now I'm going to check your breasts. You said you felt something in the left breast.

Shelly Brady Yes, that's right.

Dr Schneider About here?

Shelly Brady Yes, there.

Dr Schneider Right, I'm going to press a little bit here. Tell me if it hurts. Is that painful at all?

Shelly Brady No, that's fine.

Dr Schneider You're right, there might be something there. It might be nothing more serious than a cyst but we need to find out, so I'd like to do an ultrasound examination.

Shelly Brady Are you going to do that now?

Dr Schneider Yes, don't worry. It's only going to take a few minutes. Could you please lie down and make yourself comfortable on the examination table. I'm just going to get the ultrasound machine.

LANGUAGE

Polite instructions

The first two expressions below look rather like *if*-sentences and the last one looks like a question but actually, they are not: all three are very polite instructions or commands.

- If you'd just like to …
- If you could (just) …, that would be fine/great/ helpful …
- Could you please …?

The *going to*-future

1. **I'm going to put** this screen across.
2. **Are** you **going to do** that now?
3. Don't worry, this **isn't going to hurt**.

- Die Struktur *am/is/are going to* + Grundform des Verbs wird verwendet, um über Absichten zu sprechen (1, 2), oder wenn die Gewissheit (oder ein Anzeichen dafür) besteht, dass etwas geschehen wird (3).

3 Practice

Complete the sentences with the *going to* form of the verbs in brackets.

1. She ___ (take) a blood sample.
2. The examination ___ (not/take) very long. It's very quick.
3. ___ you ___ (give) me some medicine?
4. I ___ (press) down a little bit here.
5. How long ___ it ___ (take) to get the results?
6. You can already see she ___ (be) a difficult patient.
7. It's very busy today. They ___ (not/fit) all the patients in before lunch.
8. ___ she ___ (see) the doctor?
9. I ___ (refer) you to a radiologist.
10. ___ my symptoms ___ (get) worse?

4 Doing an ultrasound scan

Dr Schneider has found something suspicious in Shelly Brady's breast and wants to do an ultrasound scan.

LANGUAGE

Reassuring patients
There's nothing to worry about.
Please don't worry about ...
There's no need to worry/panic.
Don't worry, it's just a ...
It's just a ..., it won't hurt.
It's a very routine operation/test.
It's perfectly normal.

A Match words in the list below with the photographs.

ultrasound machine/scanner · examination table · acoustic gel · screen · pillow

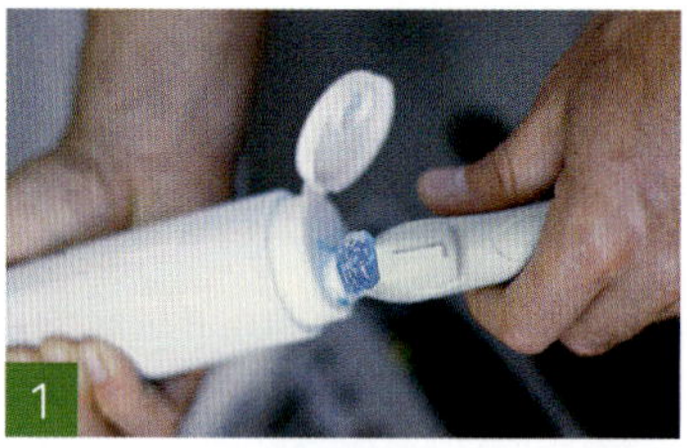
1

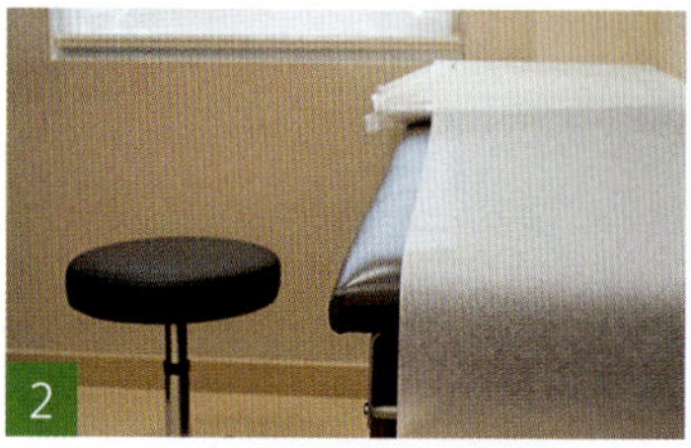
2

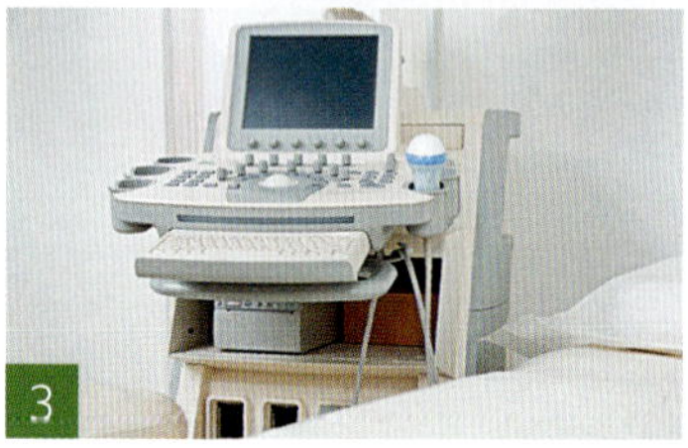
3

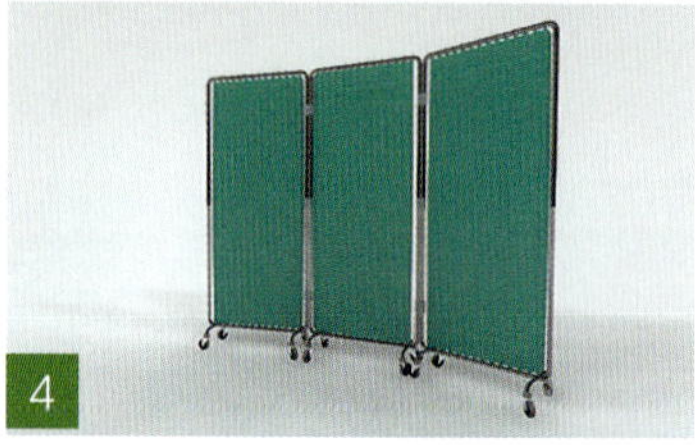
4

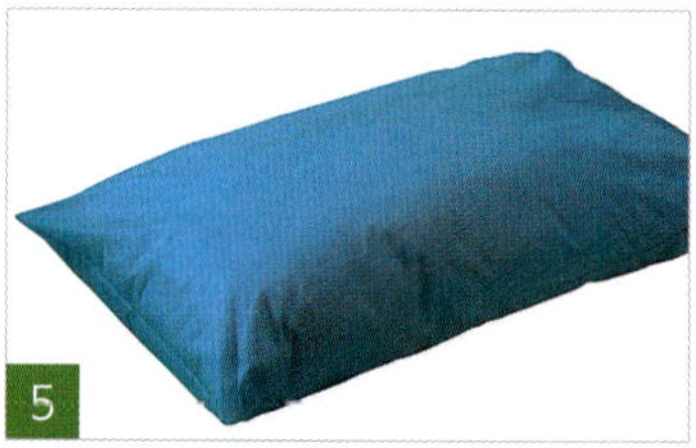
5

B 31 Listen to Dr Schneider do the scan. What is the result? Explain what action he is going to take.

C Work with a partner. Role-play a dialogue between the medical assistant and the patient.

Medical assistant

Begrüßen Sie die Patientin und beruhigen Sie sie.

Patient

Begrüßen Sie die Assistentin.

Medical assistant

Bitten Sie die Patientin sich auszuziehen und sich auf die Liege zu legen.

Patient

Fragen Sie die Assistentin, was geschehen wird.

Medical assistant

Beruhigen Sie die Patientin und erklären ihr die Abläufe.

Patient

Stellen Sie Fragen, wenn Sie etwas nicht verstanden haben.

Medical assistant

Beantworten Sie die Fragen und beruhigen Sie die Patientin.

Patient

Fragen Sie nach den Ergebnissen der Untersuchung.

Medical assistant

Erklären Sie, dass der Arzt gleich nach der Untersuchung über die Ergebnisse sprechen wird.

5 Screening for alcohol problems

Screening is also used for many other health issues. Today, you are at a training session on identifying alcohol problems. A presenter, Dr Sanders, is talking about how to screen such patients.

A 32 Listen to the presentation and complete the flow chart.

Step ①: ___ 1.

↓

STEP ②: ___ 2.
Does patient drink alcohol?
Ask when, ___ 3 and ___ 4.

→ **No heavy drinking** → Remind patients of recommended limits. Screening complete.

↓

STEP ③: ASSESS for ___ 5.
Ask patients questions about ___ 6.

→ **No serious problems** → Remind patients of recommended limits. Screening complete.

↓

STEP ④: ADVISE AND ASSIST
Tell patient they have an alcohol-use disorder.
Explain ___ 7 and agree a ___ 8.
Make a ___ 9 appointment.

↓

STEP ⑤: ___ 10.
Does patient meet drinking goal?

→ **If yes** → Continue support for at least ___ 11.

↓

STEP ⑥: Referral to ___ 12.
First recommend a ___ 13
or talk about medication.

B Work with a partner. Brainstorm and come up with some ideas for the following:

1 What reasons do you think could in fact cause alcohol-use disorder?
2 How would you define the recommended daily drink limit?
3 List some of the main health risks associated with alcohol abuse.
4 Apart from AA, what other support groups do you know of?

6 Under-age drinking

You find this article about under-age drinking on a US website.

A Work with a partner. Before you read the text, think about the situation in Germany and answer the following questions.

1 What is the minimum legal age for drinking alcohol?
2 At what age do people usually have their first experience of alcohol?
3 What are the risks of drinking alcohol as a teenager?

B Now read the text about under-age drinking in the US and compare your answers.

BINGE DRINKING

1

Alcohol is a drug. And today, like every day, more than 4,750 American kids aged 15 and younger will take their first full drink. These kids who experiment with this drug will probably consume too much alcohol over a short period of time. This is known as binge drinking. For adolescents, binge drinking means downing at least three drinks in a row for boys aged 9 to 13 or for any girl under 17. Among boys aged 14 to 15, it's four drinks.

2

Some teens drink because they have low self-esteem or think it will make them feel happier. Others are looking for new experiences. Teens also drink when many of their friends do. Girls are more likely to drink because of family problems than because of peer pressure. The problem is that many teens won't stop at a few sips. They'll binge. Normally, the liver helps remove alcohol from the blood. But when the liver cannot keep up, the alcohol then circulates through the bloodstream and brain. This is when a person becomes drunk and they can get into all kinds of trouble.

3

For instance, car accidents. One in every five teenager drivers involved in a fatal car crash has alcohol in their bloodstream. But a teenager doesn't have to be behind the wheel for alcohol to be a big risk. To begin with, binge drinkers are eight times more likely than other students to miss classes and fall behind in their work. Teens can get depressed and injure themselves, damage property or hurt someone else. Teenagers who drink are more likely to have unprotected sex, putting girls at increased risk of pregnancy and sexually transmitted diseases. Drinking can also delay puberty in girls, while abusing alcohol can cause disorders during puberty.

4

"We used to think that brain development was done by the time you're a teenager," says a research paediatrician. "Now we know that's not true. The brain keeps developing into a person's 20s and even early 30s," she explains. A new study finds that alcohol can lead to harmful changes to the brain over long periods of time. Alcohol can also hurt the so-called grey matter in a region known as the prefrontal cortex, the area used for attention, concentration, self-control and making decisions. As alcohol makes a teen less likely to turn down alcohol, the risk of binge drinking grows. This can create a cycle of inappropriate behaviour, which may lead to alcoholism in some teenagers.

C Match the headings to paragraphs 1–4.

a The dangers of binge drinking
b The causes of binge drinking
c Longer-term health risks
d What is binge drinking?

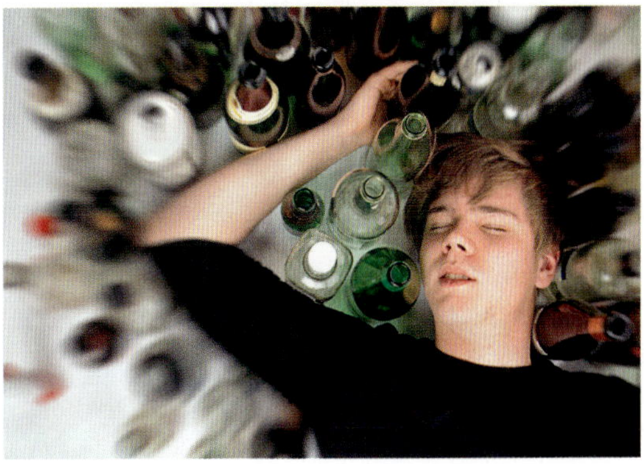

D Do the following tasks.

1. Define binge drinking.
2. Give reasons why teenagers drink alcohol, according to the author.
3. Explain what is meant by the expression 'peer pressure'.
4. Specify the differences in teenage drinking between boys and girls.
5. List the short, medium and long-term risks of drinking alcohol as a teenager.
6. Explain what is meant by a 'cycle of inappropriate behaviour'. Give some examples from your own experience.

The *will*-future

1. They think it **will make** them feel happier, but they are wrong.
2. The kids **will** probably **consume** too much alcohol.
3. They**'ll binge**, and then they**'ll injure** themselves or they**'ll hurt** someone else.
4. The problem is that many teens **won't stop** at a few sips.

- Mit *will* (+ Grundform) werden Vorhersagen und Annahmen über die Zukunft ausgedrückt, auf die wir keinen Einfluss haben. (1)
- Das *will*-Futur wird oft im Zusammenhang mit Signalwörtern wie *think, maybe, possibly* oder *probably* benutzt. (2)
- *Will* wird oft abgekürzt. (3)
- Beachte: *will not* = *won't*. (4)

7 Practice

Using the following words, make complete sentences with the correct form of *will*.

1. Teenagers – continue – to experiment with alcohol.
2. The government – not/change – the law on under-age drinking.
3. When – be – my prescription ready?
4. The drugs – help – slow down the progress of the disease.
5. A patient with a drinking problem – need – to have regular appointments.
6. The problem – not/always/get – worse quickly.
7. What kind of tests – I – have to – have?
8. When – I – get – the results of the test?

8 Practice

Complete the sentences with a suitable preposition.

1. Some teenagers turn to alcohol because ___ family problems.
2. Others simply want to experiment ___ alcohol and/or drugs.
3. The liver removes alcohol ___ the bloodstream.
4. But if there is too much alcohol for the liver to deal with, it circulates ___ the bloodstream.
5. That makes people drunk, and then they can get into all kinds ___ trouble.
6. The risk ___ binge drinking is that it can cause harmful changes ___ the brain.

9 Leseverstehen

Situation: Während Ihres Aufenthaltes in England nahmen Sie teil an einer internationalen Fachtagung zu Krebserkrankungen. In einer der Veranstaltungen, die Sie besuchten, ging es um Krebs bei Kindern und Jugendlichen. Den Teilnehmern wurde der untenstehende Text ausgehändigt.

→ Berichten Sie Ihren Kolleginnen und Kollegen von dieser Veranstaltung. Für Ihren Vortrag bereiten Sie Präsentationsfolien mit den Aussagen des Textes in englischer Sprache vor.

Cancer cases in children leap by 40% in 16 years

Fast food diets and lack of exercise could be responsible for a rise in cancer cases in young adults, scientists have warned.

Alasdair Philips, science adviser at Children with Cancer UK, says there seems to be "a correlation between the lifestyle of young people" and a significant increase in the number of teenagers being diagnosed.

"They tend to be doing a lot less exercise and there's also a lot of fast food being eaten, which is fine in moderation, but we know that it contains cancer-giving substances," he said.

"So if you eat well-cooked meat and burgers and it goes into your colon and hangs around because you're not doing much exercise, it's more likely to cause damage. I think that's part of the issue."

New analysis of official statistics by Children with Cancer UK shows how diagnosis has increased by 40% in the last 16 years, with 1,300 more cases of young people getting cancer each year.

The stark rise is most evident in colon cancer which is up by 200% and thyroid cancer which has more than doubled.

"One of the rises that has taken us a bit by surprise is this rise in colon cancer, which in the past wasn't a young person's cancer.

"Only last week the International Agency for Research on Cancer, which is part of the World Health Organization, said they'd found a relationship between obesity and too much sugar – and colon and thyroid cancer."

Children with Cancer UK says "more money and more research" is needed to examine the causes.

Around 4,000 children and young people develop cancer each year in the UK, and it is the leading cause of death in children aged one to 14.

Charlotte Hutchinson, 23, was diagnosed with leukaemia at the age of 13. She told Sky News that enduring two years of chemotherapy while trying to cope with the pressures of being a teenager was not easy.

"Obviously getting cancer at any age is never going to be easy, but as a teenager it is tough because you don't expect to get it," she said.

"As a 13/14-year-old you expect to be hanging out with your friends and just being a normal teenager – and it definitely has a knock-on effect."

10 New designer drugs

Your boss hears about new designer drugs on the radio and asks you to find out more about them. You find lots of websites on the problem including this one on a medical website. Since several of his patients are users, he is thinking about preparing a leaflet for his surgery.

Read the text then make notes in your exercise book under the following headings.

1 What are synthetic cannabinoids?
2 How are they similar/dissimilar to marijuana?
3 What symptoms do they cause?
4 Why are they so deadly?
5 Why is it so hard to control their use?

New drugs, new dangers

In the mid 1980s a team of chemists in the USA began designing a synthetic form of cannabis for research purposes. At the time, one of the chemists, John W. Huffman, said he couldn't imagine why anyone would use it for recreational purposes. Synthetic cannabis was so much more powerful and more dangerous than natural marijuana, he said, that anyone who tried it must be 'an idiot'.
The result of the work of chemists such as Huffman is a synthetic form of cannabis which can be sprayed onto natural plants to produce a huge range of new 'designer' drugs. Since the mid 2000s, hundreds of them have appeared with names such as Spice, K-2, Bliss, Blaze, Skunk or JWH-018, JWH-073 (after Huffman's initials). Each can cause a different set of severe symptoms, such as agitation, vomiting, hallucination, paranoia, seizure, chest pain, cardiac problems, stroke, kidney damage, acute psychosis, brain damage, and even death.

What are the differences to marijuana?

Marijuana contains an active ingredient called tetrahydrocannabinol (THC), which acts on the 'CB1 receptors' in the brain. CB1 receptors are in almost every part of the brain, including the central nervous system and they are normally activated by the body's own natural endocannabinoids. However, synthetic cannabinoids can be much more powerful than THC, in fact over a hundred times more. When you have a powerful and long-lasting compound affecting many different parts of the brain, the result is a range of severe effects from seizures to psychosis. The proof that synthetic cannabis is different is that an overdose with these new designer drugs is in no way the same as an overdose with natural marijuana. Marijuana users tend to be interactive, relaxed, funny. Users of synthetic cannabis, on the other hand, tend to be angry, agitated and sweat more profusely.

What are the problems of regulation?

Synthetic cannabis is not particularly difficult to make. A graduate in chemistry can easily do it. The drugs are made in secret labs in many different countries, with China in the lead. And so there is no way to check the production process or impose quality control, with the result that you just do not know exactly what you have got in your bag of Spice or K-2.
JWH was first found in Germany in 2008 – it was the JWH-018 in Spice. At first, the authorities did not know what they had found, and it took several months to have the substance analysed and identified.
As soon as they had managed this, a new compound, JWH-073, came out the following week. The producers already had it ready to sell. And now they're making something that can be bought in shops or online.

10 Applying for a job

1 The right person for the job

Work with a partner. Decide which characteristics are important for the three jobs below.

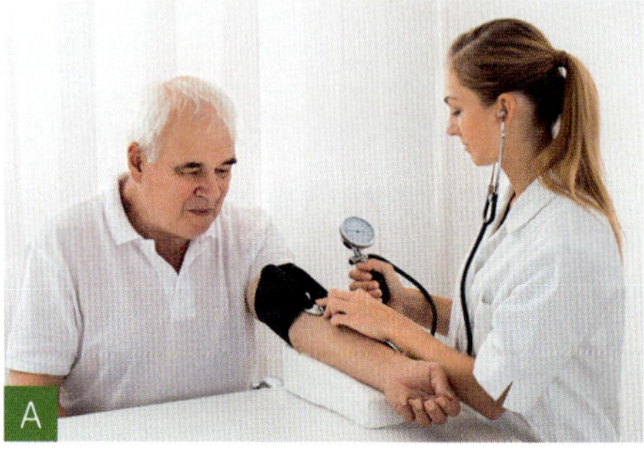

medical assistant

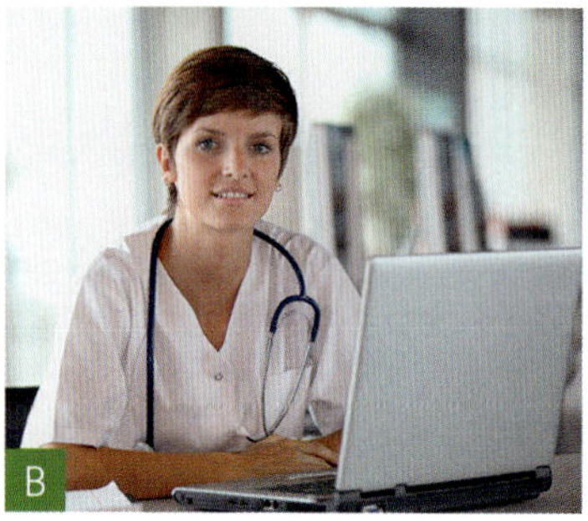

senior general practice nurse

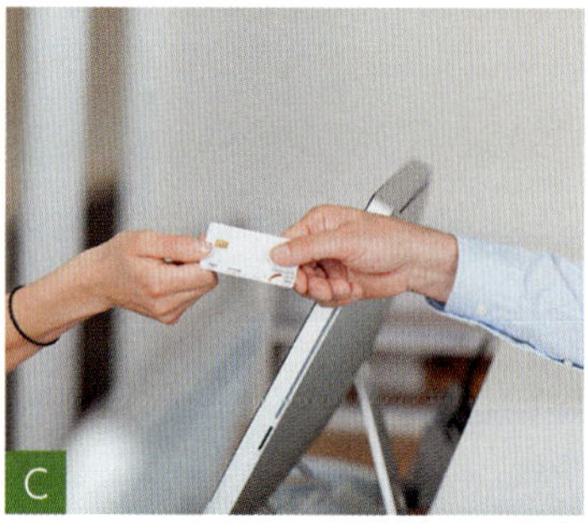

receptionist

reliable · confident · friendly · strong · talkative · quiet · cheerful · able to keep calm · a good listener · well organized · highly qualified · responsible · accurate

I think a medical assistant/ … should be ….

I agree. She/He should also be ….

A … must always be ….

I don't think a senior general practice nurse needs to be ….

Perhaps, but she/he should be ….

CULTURE

Vocational qualifications in the USA

CNA	(Certified Nursing Assistant) 75-hour vocational course.
LPN	(Licensed Practical Nurse) One-year vocational course at community colleges, technical schools or hospitals.
Certificate programs	One-year full-time courses offered by community colleges or vocational schools. Can lead to an Associate Degree Program.
Associate degree programs	Two-year full-time courses at a community college or vocational school.
RN	(Registered Nurse) Associate or full degree level qualification. A four-year college or university course. There are over 2.7m registered nurses in the USA.

CULTURE

Vocational qualifications in the UK

RN (Registered Nurse) A three-year, full-time course leading to a degree-level qualification approved by the Nursing and Midwifery Council (NMC).

FD (Foundation Degree) A two-year, full-time or three-year part-time, work-based learning programme at a university or college. Can lead to a full degree programme.

RCN (Royal College of Nursing) The largest membership organization for nurses in the UK with over 430,000 members.

GPN (General Practice Nurse) They work in GP surgeries as part of the primary healthcare team.

2 Understanding job advertisements

Ulrike is a trained German medical assistant living in the UK. She is looking for a job and finds these advertisements online.

Read the adverts and fill in the table.

Position	Duties	Qualifications	Skills	Other requirements

1 Senior Receptionist

You will be responsible for organizing our reception team. This will include work routines and dealing with both patients and staff. Minimum 5 years' experience working on reception + qualifications required. You have good organizational skills, enjoy hard work and working with a strong team. Apply to Ms Emma Trow, Nuffield House Surgery, The Meadows, Harlow, CM8 4TP.

2 Grade E Experienced Staff Nurse

Registered nurse with a minimum of three years' experience and assessment skills. Previous experience of disability assessment and experience of clinical decision-making. IT skills with experience of using a range of software. Good written and verbal communication skills and evidence of ongoing professional development. Apply to Charles Davenport, Histon Medical Centre, Histon House, Harlow CM15 7UU.

3 Care Assistant

Oak House Retirement Village requires someone with good interpersonal skills to look after elderly people. Applicants must be smart, reliable and enthusiastic about caring for people. Experience required. Apply in writing to: Sarah Mason, Oak House, High Wych Road, Sawbridgeworth, CM21 0GH.

4 Hatfield Nursing Home

We are looking for a Home Care Assistant who is 17+ with some experience of care. Applicant will look after disabled people and do a training course. Must have good people skills. Please apply in writing to:
The Manager, Hatfield Nursing Home, Chaucer Way, Hatfield, A10 6LZ.

5 Receptionist

Old Harlow Health Centre requires a receptionist for its small administration team. You will handle all inquiries, manage records and deal with patients in the waiting room. Applicants should have good communication skills, experience and good knowledge of reception software including the NHS e-Referral Service*. Apply in writing to Mrs Kay Lee, Old Harlow Health Centre, 55 Terrace Gardens, Harlow, CM18 7TQ

* The NHS e-Referral Service (ERS) is an electronic referral system used by NHS England and is designed to be a step towards achieving paperless referrals to specialists in the NHS. It allows GPs to choose the date and time of an appointment.

3 Looking for work

Three other people are looking for the job as well as Ulrike.

33 Listen to these four people talking about themselves. Which of the jobs on the previous page do you think they should apply for?

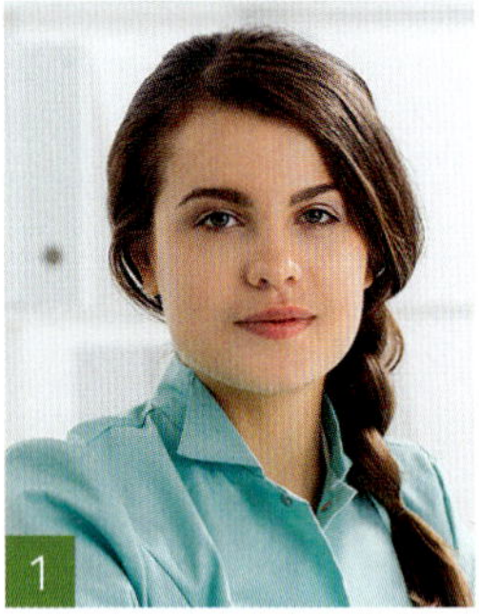
1 Ulrike

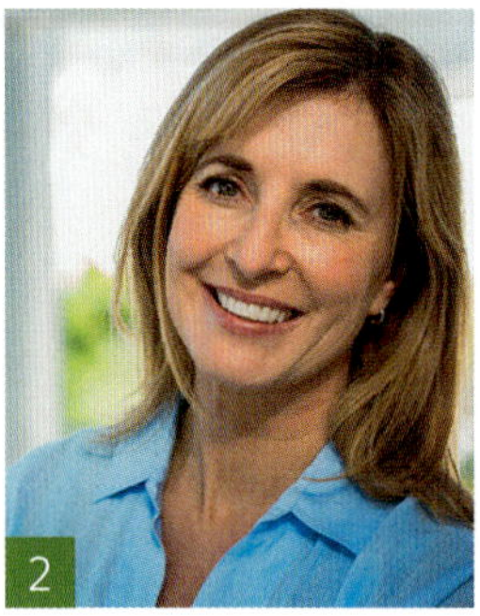
2 Sharon

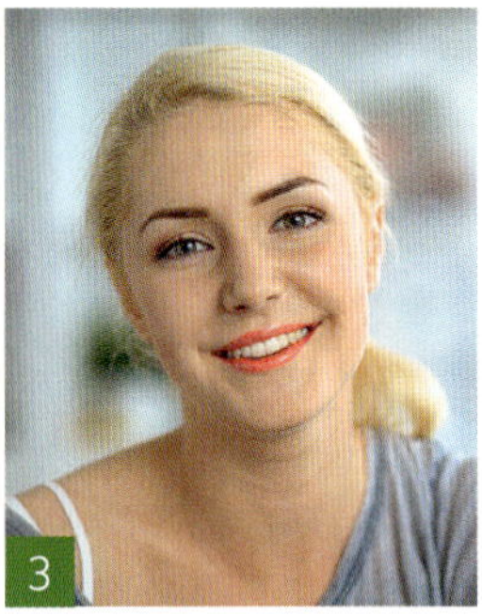
3 Kate

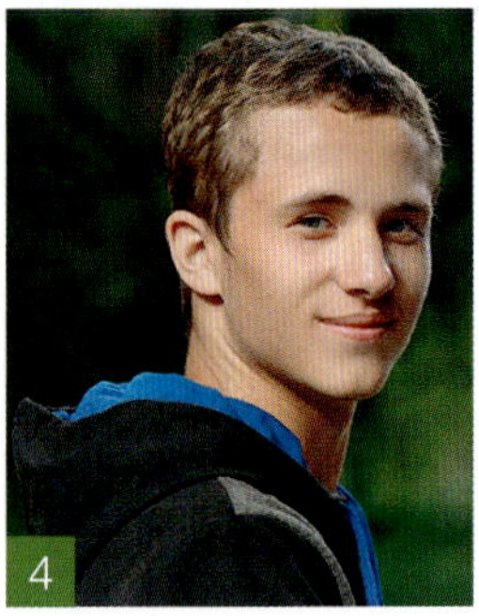
4 Tom

I think ___ should apply for the job as a ___ because ___.

4 A letter of application

Complete Ulrike's letter of application with the phrases (a–h) below.

Dear Mrs Lee

___[1] the position of receptionist which was advertised in the *Hertfordshire Evening News* of 2 June.

___[2] a shop assistant in a large department store in Harlow. ___[3] dealing with customers, offering product advice and achieving sales targets.

As you can see from my enclosed CV, ___[4] a doctor's assistant in Germany before I married and moved to the UK with my British husband. After six months I started work at John Lewis department store, where I have worked since 2014. At John Lewis ___[5] dealing with customers in an English-speaking environment.

What interested me about your advertisement was the chance to work in a small team, use some of the skills I learned during my three-year training as a doctor's assistant and to learn new skills as part of a career. I enjoy organizing information and I have excellent communication skills. ___[6] computers.

___[7] interview immediately.

___[8] hearing from you soon.

Yours sincerely
Ulrike Morris
enc.

- **a** I trained as
- **b** I am also good with
- **c** I would like to apply for
- **d** I am currently working as
- **e** I have gained experience in
- **f** I am available for
- **g** I look forward to
- **h** My duties include

5 Your curriculum vitae (CV)

Work with a partner. Make a list of all the things you should include in a good CV.

6 Writing a CV

You find an article online about writing a good CV.

A Read the article and match the headings with the paragraphs.

- a Education and professional qualifications
- b Summary
- c First impressions
- d Work experience
- e Length of CV
- f Personal details
- g Other experience

HOW TO WRITE A PROFESSIONAL CV

Your CV is a very important document; with it rest your hopes and dreams for the future – that next step up the career ladder, more money and new challenges. Your CV therefore has to represent the best you have to offer if you do not want to miss out on that perfect job you saw.

1 Your CV needs to attract the reader's attention in the first 20–30 seconds. An employer may have hundreds of CVs to look through. What an employer really wants to know is why they should invite you for an interview. If people cannot find what they want quickly, they will move on to someone else's CV. You should use appropriate headings and section breaks. Never send a hand-written CV as you will look old-fashioned and out of date.

2 It is best to try and keep your CV to a maximum of two pages of A4. If you cannot manage to do this, then you probably have not understood an employer's requirements. Employers do not want to know your whole life history – all they are interested in is enough information to decide whether they should invite you to an interview or not.

3 Always give your full name, address, mobile number and home telephone number if you have one. In the USA you don't need to include your date of birth or your marital status. You may want to include nationality if you are applying for jobs abroad.

4 List your education history, your professional qualifications and membership of professional associations. If you have recently completed a college or university degree or diploma, etc, then you may want to list the courses you studied if the subject is relevant to your target job.

5 Start with your most recent job and work backwards. Set out your main responsibilities, achievements, duties and skills that could be transferred to another employer. List your major achievements because an employer will only invite you for an interview if they can see a benefit in doing so.

6 List any computer skills you have and any foreign language skills which may be relevant for any jobs which you are applying for. Indicate whether your skills are spoken, written, business or technical.

7 List your major skills, strengths, personal qualities and achievements. Be specific, e.g. good team player, excellent written skills, versatile, able to motivate others, etc. Look at your staff appraisals or at your references for ideas.

B Say what suggestions you find surprising. Give your opinion on these suggestions.

7 A curriculum vitae (CV)

Complete Ulrike's CV with the headings below.

Qualifications • Education • Address • Date of Birth • Work Experience • Interests • Marital Status • Nationality • Additional Information

Name:	Ulrike Morris
___ 1	8 Cedar Tree Lane, Torquay, TQ1 4TR, Devon
Mobile	+44 7989 424833
Email	ulrikem2@hmail.com
___ 2	5 August 1993
___ 3	German
___ 4	Married
___ 5	2010 – 2013 Berufsschule W4 (technical college) Hamburg, Germany 2004 – 2010 Erich Kästner Gesamtschule (comprehensive school) Hamburg, Germany
___ 6	German equivalent of British GCSEs German qualification as doctor's assistant
___ 7	2014–present Shop assistant, John Lewis, Harlow Duties include dealing with customers, advising customers about products and helping the team achieve sales targets. I am also responsible for the presentation of the sales area and for managing stock levels. 2010–2013 Berufsschule W4, Hamburg Three years' work experience as a doctor's assistant in a small private practice with sandwich release for study. I passed my exams in July 2013.
___ 8	I like listening to music and going out to the theatre and cinema. I also really enjoy travelling and seeing new places.
___ 9	I am a native German speaker and have a good command of English (CEFR B2). I also speak intermediate French (CEFR A2) and have excellent computer skills. I have a full European driving licence.

8 Talking about a job application

Work with a partner. Look at Ulrike's CV, her letter of application on page 82 and the job advertisements on page 81 and answer the questions.

1 Which job did Ulrike apply for? How do you know?
2 Why is Ulrike a good candidate for the job?
3 How do her skills and qualities match the job?
4 What new skills would she have to learn?

Simple past and present perfect

1 I **married** and **moved** to the UK two years ago.
2 I **passed** my exams in July 2013.
3 She **has worked** at this department store since 2014.
4 Ulrike **has attached** her CV.
5 I **haven't written** my application yet.
6 **Have** you ever **worked** in the UK?

- Im *simple past* wird ein in der Vergangenheit vollständig abgeschlossener Vorgang geschildert. (1, 2) Es wird häufig mit einer Zeitangabe der Vergangenheit (*yesterday, last week, ago, in 2013* usw.) verwendet. (1, 2)
- Das *present perfect* wird verwendet, um auszudrücken, dass ein in der Vergangenheit begonnener Vorgang noch andauert. Dies geschieht oft in Verbindung mit Zeitbestimmungen mit *for* (+ Zeitraum) oder *since* (+ Zeitpunkt). (3)
- Das *present perfect* wird verwendet, wenn etwas in der Vergangenheit geschehen ist, das noch Auswirkungen auf die Gegenwart hat . (4) Typische Signalwörter sind *up till now, so far, just, ever already, yet.* (5, 6)
- Die Negativform wird mit *haven't/hasn't* + Partizip Perfekt gebildet. (5)
- Fragen werden mit *have/has* + Partizip Perfekt gebildet. (6)

9 Practice

Make sentences about Ulrike and use the simple past or present perfect.

1 go / to a comprehensive school in Hamburg
2 leave / school in 2010
3 after school / train as a doctor's assistant
4 gain / a lot of experience in her present job
5 not / work / for very long in Germany
6 pass / her driving test when she was 18.
7 come / to the UK in October 2014
8 Since arriving in Britain / learn to speak English very well
9 just apply / for a job in Harlow.
10 not / have / a reply from the practice yet

10 Talking about applying for a new job

Work with a partner. Use the following prompts to start a short conversation.

A: Have you seen the advert for ___?
B: No, I haven't. / Yes, I have. I saw it ___.

A: Have you finished writing your ___ yet?
B: No, I haven't. / Yes, I have. I ___ it yesterday.

A: Have you applied for ___?
B: No, I haven't. / Yes, I have. I ___ it last week.

11 Writing your CV

Look at exercise 7 on page 84 again and write your CV. Then, with a partner, compare and check.

12 Preparing for an interview

You listen to a careers adviser on the radio giving tips about how to prepare for a job interview.

34))) Listen and say which of the recommendations below the adviser gives.

- **a** Start preparing for the interview well in advance.
- **b** Find out about the company on the internet.
- **c** Make friends with people who work for the company.
- **d** Always drive to the interview.
- **e** Change your CV to match the advertisement.
- **f** Practise the interview with a friend and record it.
- **g** Buy new clothes for the interview.
- **h** Look sexy – it might help you get the job.
- **i** Have a relaxing bath on the day of the interview.
- **j** Drink lots of coffee to stay awake.

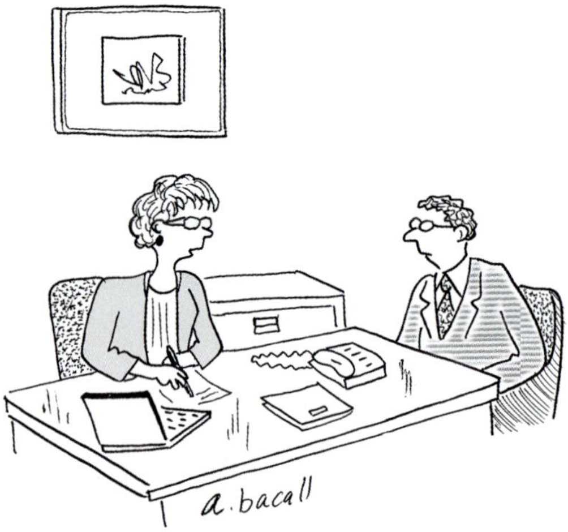

"Your MBA and PhD degrees are impressive but what concerns me is your low number of Facebook friends."

13 Practising interview questions

Here are some typical questions that you might be asked at an interview.

Work with a partner. Make interview questions and answer them.

1	where / work / at the moment	I'm working at a practice in ___.
2	how long / work / there	I've been with the practice for/since ___.
3	what / duties / include	I'm responsible for ___.
4	what / qualifications / have	I finished my training as a ___ in ___.
5	where / study	I went to ___ for three years then I ___.
6	what / hobbies and interests	I really like dancing/skydiving and ___.
7	what / enjoy / most / about /job	The thing I enjoy most about my job is ___.
8	what / strengths and weaknesses	I'm good at ___, but I'm not so good at ___.
9	why / interested in / this job	What really interested me was the ___.
10	what / relevant skills / have	My English is very good and I can ___.

LANGUAGE

Nouns ending in -er
These nouns show what the person is doing:
interviewer
trainer
employer

LANGUAGE

Nouns ending in -ee
These nouns show what is happening to the person:
interviewee
trainee
employee

14 Work with a partner

Work with a partner to prepare a job interview role-play.

- First choose one of the jobs from exercise 2 or find one on the internet in English.
- Student A is the interviewer: Prepare some questions for the candidate.
- Student B is the interviewee: Use your CV from exercise 11.

15 Interaktion: A2

Situation: You wrote an application for an internship in England and were among the lucky ones who were invited for an interview.

→ **Your assignment: Discuss the following with your partner(s):**

- You are offered an interview at 8:30 a.m. or 2 p.m. What time would you choose and why?
- How would you dress?
- What would be the first words you say when you enter the room?
- What would be your motivation for wanting an internship in the UK?
- What could you do to suppress nervousness?
- How would you prepare yourself for the interview?
- How would you deal with questions you cannot answer?
- How important is it to mention personal interests and hobbies in a job interview?

16 Produktion: B1

Situation: Sie planen ein Praktikum in einer Praxis in Großbritannien, um auch Ihre Sprachkenntnisse zu erweitern. Sie haben unten stehenden Text auf einer Internetseite gefunden.

→ **Schreiben Sie den Text eines Bewerbungsschreibens (ohne Nennung Ihres Namens, Ihrer Adresse sowie Unterschrift und Datum). Gehen Sie auf die Aspekte Patientenbetreuung, Vorbereitungsarbeiten, Büroarbeit und Sterilisation ein, indem Sie diesbezüglich jeweils zwei Ihrer Erfahrungen in diesen Bereichen schildern. Erwähnen Sie, dass Sie im Anhang einen Lebenslauf und ein kürzlich aufgenommenes Passfoto mitschicken.**

Benutzen Sie für Ihren Text diese Checkliste:

- Anrede
- Bezug auf Internetseite
- Interesse / Grund für Bewerbung
- Dauer: drei Monate
- Grafschaft Kent
- Patientenbetreuung (Erfahrung 1 und 2)
- Vorbereitungsarbeiten (Erfahrung 1 und 2)
- Büroarbeit (Erfahrung 1 und 2)
- Sterilisation (Erfahrung 1 und 2)
- Anlagen: Lebenslauf und Passfoto
- Schlusssatz

Gain knowledge and work experience in the UK

Come and join us at Internship-UK and gain the knowledge and work experience to truly set yourself apart from the crowd! Our internships are highly flexible, which means that you can pick the start and end dates of your internship.

Apply now and take the challenge to improve yourself and your knowledge by joining our team of motivated and enthusiastic interns. Launch your career today!

Please note that we require that all applicants for our internship programme have a valid UK work permit that allows them to volunteer full-time (40 hours) in the UK.

EM Extra Material

17 Working in the UK

Ulrike got the job as a receptionist and is now working at a health centre in Harlow. She is talking to a magazine reporter about the problems of working in another country.

List the things which are similar and the things which are different about training in the UK and in Germany.

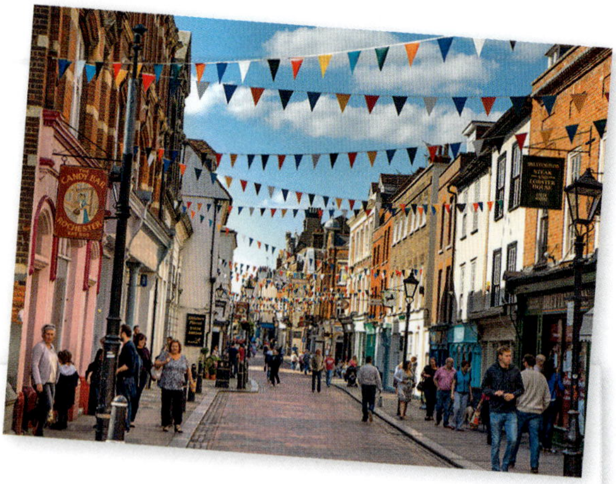

How easy was it to get a job in the UK?

Very hard! I moved here with my British husband and then had to find a job. I sent my CV to everyone – not just health centres, but also pubs, retail – it took me six months of applying for jobs and having interviews before I got my first job at a department store. It was very difficult at first because I only had school English when I came to England, so the interviews were nerve-racking!

And how did you become a receptionist?

I saw the advertisement for a receptionist and applied. I had an interview with the owner and then I talked to the girls who work here, and it just looked like a really nice place to work. And now I absolutely love it.
But I want to get back into the clinical side of general practice so I'm doing some nursing training.

What is the training like in the UK?

It's great. I'm doing an interesting two-year course in general practice nursing. The good thing is that, because of my German qualifications, I can do a lot of hours of clinical work, but, of course, I still need to pass my British exams to be a qualified nurse and to able to register with the Royal College of Nursing.

Is training in the UK very different from the training you did in Germany?

Yes and no. The clinical procedures are the same. But in Germany, as a trainee, I always felt I had little say in things and I had a senior nurse looking over my shoulder all the time. But she was very helpful and I got a good broad basic training. Here in the UK, the pay is quite good, and you get asked about changes to the practice and what you think about things.

And how do you like your job?

I absolutely love it! Every day is different and you never know what to expect.

And your future plans?

After I've qualified, I'd like to work full-time on the clinical side and not reception. Then I'd like to do a degree, I think.

18 Writing about your experience

Write about the first week in your present job and about your plans for the future.

KMK Mock Exam: B1

Schriftliche Prüfung	
Rezeption I (Hörverstehen) (20 Punkte)	*Religion forbids ...*
Rezeption II (Leseverstehen) (20 Punkte)	*Hand drying helps hand hygiene*
Produktion (30 Punkte)	E-Mail: Geburtstagsfeier für eine Ärztin
Mediation (Sprachmittlung) (30 Punkte)	Arbeitsunfähigkeitsbescheinigung
Mündliche Prüfung:	
Interaktion (30 Punkte)	Mehrere Vorschläge: *Working conditions, the waiting room, etc.*

www)) Rezeption I: Hörverstehen — Erreichbare Punkte: hier 20

Situation:
Sie arbeiten in einer großen Praxis mit internationalem Publikum. Sie sollen für Ihre Kolleginnen und Kollegen eine überschaubare Liste anfertigen, aus der hervorgeht, was Mitglieder unterschiedlicher Glaubensgemeinschaften aus religiösen Gründen nicht essen dürfen, damit sie bei der Patientenberatung nichts verkehrt machen. Sie haben bereits die untenstehende Liste mit gängigen Zutaten dafür erstellt.

In einem Blog im Internet fanden Sie zu diesem Thema ein Gespräch zwischen einem Hotelbesitzer (Doug) und einer Journalistin (Christine). Die Überschrift auf der Website besagt, dass es um Gerichte für Muslime, Hindus und Juden geht. Sie hören dieses Gespräch zweimal.

Ihre Aufgabe:
Machen Sie sich zunächst mit der untenstehenden Tabelle vertraut. Hier sollen Sie ankreuzen, welche Speisen mit den links aufgeführten Bestandteilen für welche Religion verboten sind.

	Muslims	Hindus	Jews
bacon			
beef, veal			
ham			
milk and meat products that have been in contact with each other			
pork			
shellfish			

Situation:
In Ihrer Praxis sind zurzeit fünf PraktikantInnen aus Malaysia, mit denen Sie nur auf Englisch kommunizieren können. Anscheinend haben diese über Sicherheit und Hygiene am Arbeitsplatz andere Ansichten als Sie und Ihre Kolleginnen und Kollegen, denn sie benutzen häufig nach der Handwäsche Frottierhandtücher, weil diese ihrer Meinung nach umweltschonend seien.

Ihre Aufgabe:
Um fundiert argumentieren zu können, lesen Sie den folgenden Artikel aus einer Fachzeitschrift und machen sich zu dessen Aussagen Notizen. Nutzen Sie dafür die unten stehenden Aspekte.

Hand drying helps hand hygiene

Hand hygiene is a serious matter: to eliminate microorganisms and avoid infections, you must wash your hands as if you were working in a hospital. To prevent infection, hospital guidelines advise their doctors and patients to clean their hands with care, using soap and then to dry them with paper towels. There have been many studies on the benefits of hand washing and on the effectiveness of different hand-washing soaps but relatively few on the contribution of hand drying to hand hygiene.

For effective infection control, you must also ensure that not only your hands are thoroughly clean after washing, but also that you use the most appropriate way to dry your hands. Ordinary towels are out of the question because of their low hygiene. Secondly, they are not very environmentally. friendly when one considers the amount of detergent and water required to wash them.

How else can we dry our hands and what is the most hygienic method? A study of Westminster University compared the performance of paper towels with two types of electric hand dryer: the warm-air dryer and the jet-air dryer. The two electric dryers actually increased the amount of bacteria on the hands but the paper towels reduced it.

The jet-air dryer, in particular, showed a greater potential to spread contamination to other users in the washroom and, like warm-air dryers, was liable to become contaminated with bacteria, some of which can cause disease and spread infection.

The conclusion was that single-use, paper towels beat sophisticated drying technology hands down.

Your findings concerning:
- Recommendations for people in hospitals
- The importance of hand drying
- The use of towels
- Hand-drying methods that are compared in the study
- The effects of
  - electric dryers in general
  - jet-air dryers in particular
  - paper towels

Produktion

Erreichbare Punkte: hier 30

Situation:
Während Ihres Praktikums in England wird jemand im Ärzteteam der Praxis, in der Sie arbeiten, einen „runden" Geburtstag feiern. Jeder weiß, Dr. Evelyn Zoltan mag Musik und geht häufig in die Oper und zu Konzerten.

Ihre Aufgabe:
Da es sich um eine relativ große Praxis mit vielen Mitarbeiterinnen und Mitarbeitern handelt und es schwierig ist, mit allen die Gestaltung dieses Ereignisses hinter dem Rücken von Dr. Zoltan zu besprechen, schreiben Sie eine E-Mail an Ihre Kolleginnen und Kollegen. Darin enthalten sind folgende Punkte:

- Grund für die E-Mail (runder Geburtstag)
- Art der Überraschung für diese Ärztin
- Hinweis auf Vorliebe für Musik
- Geschenk und Glückwunschkarte
- Geldsammlung dafür
- Betrag nach Belieben in die Kaffeedose in der Küche
- Bitte um Vorschlag: Ort, wo gefeiert werden soll
- Bitte um Ideen bis Ende nächster Woche an Sie per E-Mail
- Abschluss (Gruß, Dank)

Mediation

Erreichbare Punkte: hier 30

Situation:
Auf einer internationalen Tagung haben Sie eine Medizinische Fachangestellte aus den USA kennengelernt, mit der Sie sich regelmäßig per E-Mail austauschen. Gestern fragte sie bei Ihnen an, wie in Deutschland mit arbeitsunfähigen Personen umgegangen wird bzw. wie die gesetzlichen Vorgaben dafür sind. Für Ihre Auskünfte orientieren Sie sich an den Text einer Krankenkasse zu diesem Thema, den Sie im Internet fanden.

Ihre Aufgabe:
Schreiben Sie den Text einer E-Mail an Ihre amerikanische Freundin und erläutern ihr darin, welche Regelungen bei Arbeitsunfähigkeit in Deutschland existieren.

Arbeitsunfähigkeit
In Deutschland sind Arbeitnehmer/innen bei einer Erkrankung finanziell abgesichert. Ihr Arbeitgeber zahlt Ihnen für bis zu sechs Wochen Ihr Gehalt weiter, manche Tarifverträge sehen sogar noch längere Zeiträume vor. Danach haben Sie Anspruch auf Krankengeld, das Sie von der Krankenkasse erhalten. Das Krankengeld beträgt 70 Prozent des regelmäßigen Bruttoarbeitsentgelts, maximal jedoch 90 Prozent des bisherigen Nettoarbeitsentgelts. Sie erhalten es für dieselbe Krankheit maximal eineinhalb Jahre (78 Wochen).

Arbeitgeber informieren
Kann ein/e Arbeitnehmer/in aufgrund einer Erkrankung nicht zur Arbeit gehen, ist der Arbeitgeber darüber umgehend zu informieren. Welche genauen Fristen dabei einzuhalten sind und an wen man sich zu wenden hat, ist von Unternehmen zu Unternehmen anders geregelt. Informieren Sie sich deshalb bei Ihrem Arbeitgeber, um auf der sicheren Seite zu stehen. Dauert die Erkrankung länger als drei Tage, benötigen Sie in jedem Fall, unabhängig von einer speziellen Regelung bei Ihrem Arbeitgeber, eine Arbeitsunfähigkeitsbescheinigung, die von einem Arzt ausgestellt wird. Sie erhalten zwei Exemplare: eine ohne Diagnose, die für Ihren Arbeitgeber bestimmt ist; eine mit Diagnose, die Sie umgehend bei der Krankenkasse einreichen.

Die mündliche Prüfung ist eine Interaktionsprüfung zwischen mindestens zwei Kandidaten/Kandidatinnen. Sie dauert für B1 pro Kandidat/in ca. 15 min. Die Zeit, in der beide miteinander kommunizieren, zählt für beide gleichermaßen. D.h., die gesamte Prüfungsdauer kann 20-25 min dauern. Dieser zum Erwerb des KMK-Zertifikats verbindliche Prüfungsteil ist in der Regel wie folgt gegliedert:

Phase I: Die Kandidaten/Kandidatinnen berichten individuell darüber, warum sie sich für diesen Beruf entschieden haben, über ihre bisherigen beruflichen Tätigkeiten (Vorlieben/Abneigungen) bzw. über ihre berufliche Laufbahn, Pläne und Wünsche. Die Kandidaten/Kandidatinnen werden im Wechsel befragt.

Phase II (Interaktionsphase 1) ggf. mit Vorbereitungszeit, abhängig von der Komplexität der Aufgabenstellung: Es sollte sich vorrangig um Expertengespräche handeln, weniger um Gespräche zwischen Patienten/Patientinnen. Das kann bedeuten, dass beide bzw. alle Kandidaten/Kandidatinnen die gleichen Materialien vorliegen haben. Im Folgenden geht es um Gestaltungsmöglichkeiten dieser Phase.

Phase III (Interaktionsphase 2): Beispielsweise mit dem Auftrag: „In Part Three both / all of you are going to evaluate a photo / a graph / a website."

Ihre Aufgaben für Phase I könnten wie folgt lauten:

Geben Sie Auskünfte über sich und Ihren beruflichen Werdegang anhand folgender Stichworte:

- Your professional career:
  - Training, qualifications, internships etc.
  - Reasons why you chose this job / career path
- The practice/institution:
  - General practice or one with a field of specialization
  - Number of physicians/employees
  - Equipment
  - Working conditions
- Your experiences / daily routine in the practice/institution:
  - Administrative tasks (give examples)
  - Medical tasks (give examples)
  - Your likes/dislikes

Ihre Aufgaben für Phase II könnten wie folgt lauten:

Situation:
Sie unterhalten sich während Ihres Praktikums in London mit einer Kollegin über eines der unten aufgeführten Themen. Geben Sie stets Begründungen für Ihre Argumente oder Beispiele:

- What qualities must a healthcare assistant have? Which ones are the most important?
- How important do you consider the following items in the waiting room?
  - Choice of magazines
  - Drinks (such as cooled water)
  - Children's toys/corner
  - Room design: pictures on the wall, wallpaper, posters
- Should there be a dress code for employees?
- As regards your work experience, what suggestions can you make to improve working conditions? (Think about working hours, breaks, facilities, etc.)
- What are the essential elements for a good website for a practice/institution?
- Patients often show their appreciation by putting money in a small box at reception. Would you prefer sweets/chocolate or a handshake or just a "thank you" instead?

Transcripts

Track 3: Unit 1, Exercise 6A

Joanna	Good morning. Ashbrook Health Centre. Can I help you?
Patient	Good morning. Yes, I've got an appointment with you later today. Can you tell me how to get to the centre, please?
Joanna	Sure, how are you getting here?
Patient	That's why I'm calling. What's the best way to get to you?
Joanna	OK, it's easy to get here by underground, train or car.
Patient	I'm not sure yet how I'll be coming, so if I come by train ...
Joanna	OK, then the nearest station is Upper Holloway. It's very close to us. You come out of the train station onto a main road, called Holloway Road. Go left on Holloway Road and then you take the first right into Fairbridge Road. Go straight on for about 300 metres and then turn left into Ashbrook Road. We are on the left, on the corner of St John's Villas, number 56.
Patient	OK, thanks. You said there was an underground station nearby, too.
Joanna	Yes, it's Archway and it's on the Northern Line. The station is on a big roundabout on Holloway Road. You turn right on Holloway Road heading south – don't go down Junction Road – and then take your second left into Elthorne Road. Again, after about three hundred metres, turn right into Ashbrook Road, and we're on the corner of Ashbrook Road and St John's Villas. It's only a 5-minute walk.
Patient	That's great, thanks. And if I want to go by car?
Joanna	If you are coming from the north, go over the roundabout at Archway and just drive down Holloway Road. You can't take the second left into Elthorne Road because it's a one-way street, so take the third left into St John's Villas and we are on the corner at the end of the road, number 56. We don't have any parking at the centre, so you have to park on the street, I'm afraid, and it can be difficult to find a parking spot sometimes.
Patient	OK, thanks. See you later.
Joanna	No problem. See you later. Goodbye.

Track 5: Unit 2, Exercise 3

Narrator	Phone call number 1.
Sarah	So, your appointment's on Wednesday at eleven thirty, Mrs Nicholl. That's half past eleven on the 25 June.
Narrator	Phone call number 2.
Sarah	That's right, Mrs Hanson, your appointment's now on Friday at four fifteen, that's quarter past four.
Narrator	Phone call number 3.
Sarah	Hello, Mr Watts. You can have an appointment next Tuesday at ten to twelve. All right? Great. So, that's eleven fifty on Tuesday 20 April.
Narrator	Phone call number 4.
Sarah	I'm sorry, Mr Thomas. I'm afraid the only appointment I have is at a quarter to nine.
Narrator	Phone call number 5.
Sarah	Hello, Mrs Dobson. I'm sorry but we can't fit you in at 8:30 – we can only do 9:30.

Track 6: Unit 2, Exercise 4

Narrator	Phone call number 1.
Sarah	Good morning, Epping Health Centre. Can I help you?
Mrs Taylor	Hello. My name's Mrs Taylor, I'd like to make an appointment, please .
Sarah	Certainly, is there any particular day or time you would prefer?
Mrs Taylor	Yes, is Thursday OK? In the morning?
Sarah	We can do Thursday at eight forty if that's OK?
Mrs Taylor	That's great, thanks.
Sarah	OK, Mrs Taylor, see you on Thursday.
Narrator	Phone call number 2.
Sarah	Good morning, Epping Health Centre. Can I help you?
Mr Hall	Yes, Mr Hall here, I'd like to make an appointment, please.
Sarah	Certainly, Mr Hall, is there any particular day or time you would prefer?
Mr Hall	Yes, Thursday, late morning, please.
Sarah	We can do Thursday at ten past eleven if that's OK?
Mr Hall	That's great, thanks.
Sarah	OK, Mr Hall, see you on Thursday.
Narrator	Phone call number 3.
Sarah	Good morning, Epping Health Centre. Can I help you?
Mrs Marsh	Hi, it's Sandra Marsh. Can I make an appointment, please?
Sarah	Certainly, is there any particular day or time you would prefer, Mrs Marsh?
Mrs Marsh	Yes, I can do Thursday afternoon. Is that OK?
Sarah	Let's see. We can do ten to two in the afternoon?
Mrs Marsh	That's great, thanks.
Sarah	OK, Mrs Marsh, see you on Thursday.
Narrator	Phone call number 4.
Sarah	Good afternoon, Epping Health Centre. Can I help you?
Mrs Hiley	Good afternoon, I'd like to make an appointment, please.
Sarah	Certainly, is there any particular day or time you would prefer?
Mrs Hiley	Yes, is Thursday afternoon OK?
Sarah	I'm afraid we're very busy in the afternoon. Can you do half past eleven?
Mrs Hiley	Err, OK. That's fine.
Sarah	Good. Can I have your name, please?
Mrs Hiley	Oh yes, it's Hiley, Susan Hiley. That's H-I-L-E-Y.
Sarah	Thanks, Mrs Hiley. See you on Thursday.

Track 7: Unit 2, Exercise 7

Narrator	Name number 1.
Man	Could I have your name, please?
Mrs Gawlinski	Yes, it's Gawlinski. That's G-A-W-L-I-N-S-K-I.

Man	Thank you, Mrs Gawlinski. And could I have your …

Narrator	Name number 2.
Mr Tuncay	Good morning. My name is Tuncay. I have an appointment for 10.30.
Woman	Could you spell that please, Mr Tuncay?
Mr Tuncay	It's T-U-N-C-A-Y.
Woman	Ah, yes. Here you are. Please take a seat, Mr Tuncay.

Narrator	Name number 3.
Man	Could you please spell your name, Mr Kuznetsov?
Mr Kuznetsov	Yes, it's K-U-Z-N-E-T-S-O-V.
Man	That's great. Thank you, Mr Kuznetsov.

Narrator	Name number 4.
Woman	How do you spell your name, Mr Yildirim?
Mr Yildirim	It's Y-I-L-D-I-R-I-M.
Woman	Right. Thank you, Mr Yildirim.

Narrator	Name number 5.
Woman	So, that's Wysocki spelt W-I-Y-S-O …
Mrs Wysocki	No, it's spelt W-Y-S-O-C-K-I.
Woman	Oh, I am sorry. Thank you, Mrs Wysocki.

Narrator	Name number 6.
Man	I'm sorry but can you tell me how to spell your name please, Mrs Leigh?
Mrs Leigh	Sure. It's L-E-I-G-H.
Man	Thank you very much, Mrs Leigh.
Mrs Leigh	You're welcome.

Track 8: Unit 2, Exercise 12

Good morning, this is Elizabeth Graham. I hope you remember me. I was at the practice last Tuesday. My next appointment is tomorrow at half four, but I'm awfully sorry but I have to cancel because my cellar is flooded due to the heavy rain last night, and I have to be at home when the workmen come to sort things out. So, could you please make a new appointment for me at the end of next week? That would really good. My telephone number is 6776993 (six – double seven – six – double nine – three). Oh and yes, before you call, could you please do me a favour and check the umbrella stand in the waiting room? I think I perhaps left mine there. It's my favourite umbrella, you see. It's red, white and blue. Yes, that's right – the colours of the Union Jack. Thank you very much. Have a nice day.

Track 9: Unit 2, Exercise 13

First caller

Good morning, this is Elizabeth Graham. I hope you remember me. I was at the practice last Tuesday. My next appointment is tomorrow at half four, but I'm awfully sorry but I have to cancel because my cellar is flooded due to the heavy rain last night, and I have to be at home when the workmen come to sort things out. So, could you please make a new appointment for me at the end of next week? That would really good. My telephone number is 6776993 (six – double seven – six – double nine – three). Oh and yes, before you call, could you please do me a favour and check the umbrella stand in the waiting room? I think I perhaps left mine there. It's my favourite umbrella, you see. It's red, white and blue. Yes, that's right – the colours of the Union Jack. Thank you very much. Have a nice day.

Second caller

Good afternoon. Oh, I forgot today is a public holiday in Germany. I hope you'll listen to your voicemail on Wednesday morning and ring me back because this is rather urgent. My name's Wanda Turnbull – that's W – A – N – D – A – T – U – R – N – B – U – double L. I'm on a business trip and I'm staying at the Hotel Schwarzenberg until Friday. The receptionist recommended Dr. Rose to me and gave me a card with his telephone number and address. I'm calling because I've just come off a 32-hour flight from Sydney with various stopovers and I'm pretty shattered. And, as you can no doubt imagine, I'm suffering from jetlag and simply can't concentrate! And unfortunately, I forgot to have my B12 injection before I left.
As I have to give a presentation in front of rather a lot of people on Thursday morning, I would like to look fresh and relaxed for my audience. Besides, my talk will be videoed, and so that's another reason why I want to look my best. So, I hope you can squeeze me in. Any time on Wednesday would suit me. I would be most grateful if you could phone me back at the hotel. The number is 43 11 06 – extension 233 (four – three – double one – oh – six, extension two – double three).
And yes, I have private health insurance – I'm from Australia – and will settle my bill straightaway by credit card or in cash. I hope you can call me as soon as possible. Thank you very much.

Track 10: Unit 3, Exercise 3A

1

Kerstin	Guten Morgen. Kann ich Ihnen behilflich sein?
Adnan	Can you speak English?
Kerstin	Yes. Can I help you?
Adnan	I have a very bad pain in my chest. I need to see a doctor.
Kerstin	When did the pain start?
Adnan	It started this morning.
Kerstin	Can you breathe normally?
Adnan	No, I had problems walking up the stairs just now. I couldn't breathe very well …

2

Kerstin	Hallo, es geht gleich los. Moment, bitte.
Zeynap	Do you speak English?
Kerstin	Yes, I do but just wait a moment, please. (waits) OK, so, how can I help you?
Zeynap	My mother is sick. She's at home in bed. She's very old and has a fever. Can the doctor come to the house and see her?
Kerstin	Where do you live?
Zeynap	In Stresemannstraße. It's not very far from here …

3

Kerstin	Einen schönen guten Morgen. Wie kann ich Ihnen helfen?
Karolina	Do you speak English?
Kerstin	Yes, I do.
Karolina	Oh good. Well, my daughter spilled some boiling water on her arm and she's in a lot of pain. Can I see the doctor?
Kerstin	When did it happen?
Karolina	It happened about an hour ago. I put some cold water on it, but she said it hurt too much to put any clothes over her arm and she is still crying.
Kerstin	Can I see her arm? Hmm. That looks very red still and very sore …

4

Kerstin	Guten Tag. Kann ich Ihnen helfen?
Gianna	Do you speak English?

Kerstin Yes, I do. Can I help you?
Gianna Yes, I hurt my foot at work today. It's very painful. Can I see the doctor?
Kerstin When did it happen?
Gianna It happened when I got to work this morning, when I got out of my car. I slipped on some ice on the path.
Kerstin Can you walk on it OK?
Gianna Yes, but it hurts when I do.
Kerstin Is it swollen?
Gianna Yes, a bit.
Kerstin Did you put any ice or something cold on it?
Gianna No, I didn't put anything on it. I had a meeting I had to go to …

5
Kerstin Guten Morgen. Wie kann ich Ihnen helfen?
Paul Do you speak English?
Kerstin Yes. How can I help you?
Paul Yes, I'm taking some antibiotics at the moment but they ran out this morning. Can I get another prescription, please? I still have a bit of a cough …

Track 11: Unit 3, Exercise 3C

1
Kerstin Please take a seat. I'll ask the doctor to see you as soon as he is free.

2
Kerstin Could I take your details, please? We can then make an appointment for a home visit.

3
Kerstin Can I see her arm? Hmm. That looks very red still and very sore … I'm afraid the doctor's out visiting a patient at the moment, so I think you should go to A&E at the hospital straightaway.

4
Kerstin I'm afraid you'll have to make an appointment, and we're full today. Can you come back in the morning?

5
Kerstin I'm afraid the doctor will need to see you before he can give you a repeat prescription. Can you give me your details, so we can make an appointment …?

Track 12: Unit 3, Exercise 7A

Sarah Mr Singh? Mr Singh? Ah, hello. Dr Alexander can see you now. It's treatment room 2. Go through the doors here and it's the room in front of you.
Man Here's the key to the patients' toilets, Mrs Watson. Just go through the doors here and turn left. Go down the corridor and then turn left again and the toilets are on your right.
Sarah Mrs Anderson. Will you go to treatment room 3, please? That's through the doors here and then turn left. Go down the corridor and then it's the third door on your right. It's right at the end of the corridor.
Man Hello. Are you from Harlan Medical Supply Company? Can you show me your ID card, please? Thank you. Let me see the delivery note, please. Ah, yes. Six boxes with supplies for the laboratory. Could you take them to the lab, please? The nurse there will check everything and sign the delivery note. Go through the doors here and turn left. Go along the corridor and then left again and it's the third door on your right. Thank you.
Sarah Hello, Mrs Compton from Fife Pharmaceutical Company? Can I see your ID card, please? That's fine, thanks. Dr Bradley is waiting for you in the office. Go through the doors here and then turn left. Go along the corridor and turn left again. It's the room at the end of the corridor.
Man Mr Samuels? Please go to the X-ray room, Mr Samuels. That's through the doors here and then turn left. Go down the corridor and turn left. The X-ray room is the first room on your left.

Track 13: Unit 3, Exercise 10A and 10B

John Good morning, Saxon Office Supplies. Can I help you?
Emily Yes, I'd like to make an order, please.
John OK, great. Do you have a customer reference number?
Emily Yes, it's 235432.
John And could I have the first line of your address, please?
Emily It's the Lea Valley Health Centre.
John And could I have your name, please?
Emily It's Emily Watson.
John OK, Emily, my name's John. What would you like to order?
Emily I'd like some Post-It notes, please. The large ones. Do you have any packs with different colours?
John So that's the 76 x 127 size. They're in packs of 12. Ah, we don't have any of the coloured packs at the moment, I'm afraid. Only the yellow ones. Is that OK?
Emily That's fine. Can I have three packs, please?
John Of course. That's three packs at £18.99 each.
Emily I need some staples, too. The 26/6 ones.
John OK, they come in boxes of 5000 and cost £2.50 each. How many would you like?
Emily Five boxes, please. And I need some pens, too. Do you have any of those ballpoint Supergrip pens? Blue ones, please.
John We only have two boxes of the blue ones left, I'm afraid. Would you like any of the black ones? They're both £4.70 for a box of five.
Emily No, it's OK. Just the two blue ones, thanks.
John OK, anything else?
Emily Yes, one last thing. I need some HP364 printer cartridges. Do you have any of the XL size?
John One moment, 364 … we do, yes. Which colours do you need?
Emily Do you have a pack with all four colours?
John We do, in fact, they're on special offer this week – £45.50 for a pack of four.
Emily Oh, that's good. Then, two packs please, and that's everything.
John Great, OK, so all together that comes to, let me see, …

Track 14: Unit 3, Exercise 13

MFA OK, so now I have some more questions for you. Are you having any kind of medical treatment at the moment?
Sarah No, I'm not.
MFA Have you ever had an allergic reaction to any kind of treatment before? You know, to drugs, injections or an anaesthetic, for example.
Sarah No, I haven't.

MFA Are you taking medication at the moment? If so, what?
Sarah Err, no I'm not. No.
MFA Are you pregnant?
Sarah Yes, I am. I'm three months pregnant.
MFA OK, so that's three months pregnant. And the next question … Are you HIV positive?
Sarah No. I'm not.
MFA And when did you last see a doctor?
Sarah I haven't been to see a doctor for about a year.
MFA And do you have any health problems at the moment?
Sarah No, I don't.
MFA OK. Do you have hepatitis B?
Sarah No.
MFA OK, and finally, do you get anxious when receiving medical treatment?
Sarah Well, I do get a bit nervous about injections, yes.

Track 15: Unit 4, Exercise 2A

Sandra Hello, good morning Mr Jarvis. My name's Sandra Waterman. How are you today?
Ron Very well, thanks.
Sandra Is this your first visit to our practice?
Ron Yes, it is. I moved to the town three months ago.
Sandra Oh really? And where did you live before?
Ron In a small village called Shepton, about six miles away.
Sandra Oh, I know Shepton very well. It's a pretty place, isn't it?
Ron Yes, it is. Very.
Sandra Now, can you hold this tray for me under your ear?
Ron Yes, I can, sure.
Sandra That's great, thanks. And who was your GP there?
Ron I went to Dr Wheeler at the Maltings Health Centre.
Sandra Oh yes, Dr Wheeler's very nice. I lived in Shepton for five years, but I didn't work at the Maltings.
Ron Where did you work?
Sandra I worked here! Now I'm going to start syringing your ear. Tell me if it hurts at all, OK? Right, here we go. I moved here fifteen years ago but I began working here twenty years ago.
Ron That's a long time! Did you always want to be a nurse?
Sandra Yes, I did. I knew I wanted to be a nurse when I was still at school.
Ron So, did you leave school and start your training straightaway?
Sandra Yes, I did. And then this was the first job I applied for. Is this comfortable for you? It isn't painful at all?
Ron No, it isn't, it's fine. I think I can hear better already!

Track 16: Unit 4, Exercise 4A and 4B

Right, so that's the ear finished. Now the next part of what we call ENT – or ear, nose and throat – is of course the nose, together with the mouth and the throat. So, if you look in your books at page 32, you can see a diagram of the nose, mouth and throat.

Let's begin with the nose. First of all you have the nasal passage at the start of the nose. This is the most important passage for taking air into the body. As air goes through the nasal passage, it passes over the olfactory nerves and these send information about smell to the brain. The air then goes down into the back of the mouth, into the throat and then into the trachea – or windpipe, which carries the air to the lungs.

Now if we look at the mouth, we can see the teeth and the lips at the front and then in the middle of the mouth we can see the palate, which is the roof of the mouth, and the tongue, which is of course, the major organ of taste. But remember, smell is also an important part of the way we taste things. Anyway, when we eat or drink, the food goes from the mouth into the back of our throats and when we swallow, it goes into our gullet – or oesophagus –, which is the tube that carries food into the stomach.

Track 17: Unit 4, Exercise 9B

Nurse Mr Carr. You and your son Stephen can see Dr Scott now.
Dr Scott Hello, Mr Carr. Hello, Stephen. Now then. What's the problem?
Mr Carr Hello, Dr Scott. My son Stephen says his ear hurts. He didn't sleep at all last night and I think he has got a temperature.
Dr Scott Well, let's take a look. Stephen, I'd like you to …

Nurse Mrs Taylor? You can go in now. Dr Scott is ready for you.
Dr Scott Good afternoon, Mrs Taylor. You don't look very well today.
Mrs Taylor I feel terrible, Dr Scott. I keep sneezing, my nose is blocked, but keeps running and I also keep coughing a lot. I don't really feel tired, I just want my nose to stop running.
Dr Scott I'd like you to open your mouth and say …

Nurse Mr Tuncay? Please go in. Dr Scott will see you now.
Dr Scott Please sit down, Mr Tuncay.
Mr Tuncay Thank you, Dr Scott. I really don't feel very well.
Dr Scott Can you describe your symptoms?
Mr Tuncay Yes, I think I have a temperature. I feel really tired and my arms and shoulders ache. And my nose keeps running, and I have a sore throat.
Dr Scott Do you cough at all?
Mr Tuncay Yes, quite often.
Dr Scott I see. Please take off your shirt, Mr Tuncay. I'd like to …

Nurse You can go in now, Mrs Anderson.
Dr Scott Hello, Mrs Anderson. Please sit down and tell me what's wrong.
Mrs Anderson Hello, Dr Scott. I feel terrible. My stomach is really painful and I keep vomiting and I have a fever. I keep feeling hot and then cold.
Dr Scott Do you have diarrhoea, as well?
Mrs Anderson Yes, I do.
Dr Scott When did all this start, Mrs Anderson?
Mrs Anderson Well, I first noticed that I had a temperature last …

Nurse Hello, Mrs Morris. You and your daughter can go in now.
Dr Scott Hello, Mrs Morris. And who is this pretty little girl?
Mrs Morris This is Lucy, Dr Scott. Say hello to Dr Scott, Lucy. Sorry, she's very shy.
Dr Scott Never mind. Could you describe your daughter's symptoms, Mrs Morris?
Mrs Morris Yes, Lucy says she has a headache and doesn't feel well. I took her temperature and I think she has a fever. She also has a rash of small, red spots on her chest. Her nose keeps running and she has a bit of a cough, as well.

Dr Scott OK, Mrs Morris, I'd like you to bring Lucy over here. I'd like to take a look at that rash first. And then I'd like to ...

Track 18: Unit 4, Exercise 11A

Nurse Mr Carter. The doctor can see you now.
Andrew Carter Oh, great.
Nurse It's treatment room three. The one on the right.
Andrew Carter OK. Thanks.
Dr Scott Good morning, Mr Carter. What's the problem?
Andrew Carter I've cut my arm, doctor.
Dr Scott OK. Then let's take a look at it. Could you roll up your sleeve, please?
Andrew Carter Sure.
Dr Scott That's better. Hmm. When did this happen?
Andrew Carter This morning. I was trying to take the chain off my bike. I was using a screwdriver and it slipped. I cleaned the cut and put a bandage on it.
Dr Scott Well, you did the right thing. It's a long cut, but it isn't very deep. And it's very clean and should heal quickly. Don't worry, it will only need two or three stitches. Have you had a tetanus injection recently?
Andrew Carter I had one five or six years ago, but I can't remember when exactly.
Dr Scott Well, you'll need a tetanus injection.
Andrew Carter OK.
Dr Scott But first I'll clean and disinfect the cut before I start with the stitches. Just hold out your arm, Mr Carter and ...

Track 19: Unit 5, Exercise 2B

Dr Müller So, Mr Gray, this is going to sting a bit.
Mr Gray Ouch!
Dr Müller I'm just cleaning the wound before I start stitching. That all looks good – nice and clean. Do you have the hypodermic, please, Kerstin? Thanks. I'm giving you a local anaesthetic now, Mr Gray, so you won't feel the stitches.
Mr Gray OK, thanks.
Dr Müller It'll take a minute or two for the anaesthetic to take effect. I'll be back in a moment.
Hello again, Mr Gray, how are you doing? While Kerstin is getting everything ready, I'm going to just clean the wound again. There we are. Ready?
Mr Gray Yes.
Dr Müller Good. If you wish, you can look away while I'm doing the stitches.
Mr Gray That's a good idea, I think I will.
Dr Müller No problem. I'm just starting the first stitch now. It doesn't hurt, does it?
Mr Gray No. I can feel that you are doing the stitches, but it doesn't hurt.
Dr Müller That's good. Nearly there. I'm just finishing off the last one. And now I am tying off the stitches. There we are.
Kerstin, could you please dress the wound? Thank you.
Kerstin OK, Mr Gray, this won't take very long. There we are, nearly done. I think it's safe for you to look again.
Mr Gray OK, thanks.
Dr Müller I'll leave Kerstin to finish off, and we'll see you in a few days.

Track 20: Unit 5, Exercise 4

Mary Good morning. I'm Mary Smith and I have an appointment for a blood test and an immunization for hepatitis A.
Kerstin Oh yes. Good morning, Mrs Smith. I'll take you straight to the treatment room. It's along here on the left. Here we are. Please wait here, and I'll tell Dr Müller that you are here and waiting for your immunization.
Mary OK, thanks.
Kerstin Here I am again, Mrs Smith. I can take the blood sample while we're waiting for Dr Müller. Could you take off your jacket and roll up your sleeve, please?
Mary Is that high enough?
Kerstin That's fine. Now, I'm just putting on a tourniquet before I take the sample. Does that feel OK? Not too tight?
Mary No, that's fine.
Kerstin Good. And now the needle. This might hurt a little bit – but not much. There we are. That's it. Now I'll take the blood sample. Best to look away, Mrs Smith. Lots of people don't like the sight of blood. There – I'm finished. That didn't take long, did it? Now I can take off the tourniquet, take out the needle and we're done.
Mary Great. I'm glad that's over!
Kerstin Yes, the worst is over. Could you just hold this cottonwool swab on your arm for a minute or two, please?
Mary Sure.
Kerstin Right. I'll put a plaster on and then we're done. Please wait here, Mrs Smith. Dr Müller will be with you in a minute or two for the immunization. OK?
Mary Yes, thank you.

Track 21: Unit 6, Exercise 1A

Mike I'm Mike Sheffield and this is my daughter, Shelley. She's here for a smallpox vaccination. I've told her that it won't hurt, but she's still anxious. A doctor's practice is a scary place for a young kid.

Susan My name is Susan Farrows. I'm 16 and I'm here for a pelvic examination. I've never had a pelvic examination before and I'm feeling a bit nervous.

Rachel I'm Rachel Monahan. I really just want to renew my prescription medication. Normally I just phone in and the doctor sends it to me by post, but this time the doctor wants to take some blood and urine samples first. My husband has taken a day off work so that he can drive me here and then pick me up later and take me home.

Li My name is Yao Li and I'm from Canton. I'm a student here. I was at the beach with some friends and I cut my foot on a broken bottle. It isn't a serious cut, but I think I should have a tetanus injection.

Barney I'm Barney Redford. I've got an awful pain in my back. I haven't been here for a couple of years. I don't like going to the doctor's. You have to sit in a waiting room with people coughing and spreading their germs. You never know what diseases they might have.

Track 22: Unit 6, Exercise 6A and 7A

Nurse Doctor, that was great the way you dealt with that nervous patient.

Dr Graham Thank you. Do you know, I've been a doctor now for nearly 30 years and the patients still have the same old fears as when I started!

Nurse How do you mean?

Dr Graham Well, medicine has changed so much in the last 30 years but people still fear the same things. Take injections, for example, a lot of people still get really nervous about getting injections – everyone remembers how painful they were as a kid – but now we use smaller needles and make sure that giving an injection or taking blood is as comfortable and painless as possible.

Nurse I remember my doctor when I was a kid. He was really scary!

Dr Graham I know. And 30 years ago doctors weren't expected to spend so much time with their patients. We're all told now that we should spend more time talking to our patients and listening to them, and we should always explain the risks and the benefits of each treatment. I suppose if it means patients don't feel so helpless and anxious, then it's a good idea.

Nurse But not all doctors are friendly like you, Dr Graham.

Dr Graham Well, I try, but like many doctors, I don't really have much more time for my patients now than doctors had thirty years ago. And I guess some doctors today think that progress in diagnosis and medication means that they don't have to talk to their patients! But the patient has got to trust you or they shouldn't start the treatment. And the instruments! In the old days, they used to be really big and scary!

Nurse But instruments nowadays are much smaller. Many instruments are now digital and less invasive.

Dr Graham That's right. And they worry that we're too busy and don't have time to do our job properly – so we need to make a relaxed atmosphere and not look rushed.

Nurse And I bet they didn't have TVs in the waiting room when you started!

Dr Graham That's true! Or soft music playing in the surgery ... I know a doctor who burns aromatherapy candles in his office ...

Nurse No! I even read about one who gave foot spas and massages in his surgery!

Dr Graham I think that's going a bit far! I'm sure the patients all love these things, but I don't think they really relieve anxiety any better than simply listening to the patient and explaining what you're doing!

Track 23: Unit 6, Exercise 11

Susan Er, hallo? I've got an appointment for 10.30.

Meike Ah, yes. Here we are, Miss Farrows. It's Susan, isn't it?

Susan Yes, that's right.

Meike And you're here for a pelvic exam. Is this your first one?

Susan Er, yes, it is.

Meike OK. Please follow me. I'll take you to a treatment room. There's nothing to worry about. It won't hurt at all. Here we are. Now, before the doctor comes, I need to measure your blood pressure. Please take your jacket off, Susan, and roll up the sleeve of your right arm. That's it, thank you. OK. Your blood pressure is a little high today. Are you nervous, Susan?

Susan A bit, yes.

Meike There's nothing to be nervous about, it's just a routine check-up. Do you know what happens in the exam?

Susan Not really, no. That's why I'm a bit nervous.

Meike It's OK, that's normal the first time. Well, when you see the doctor he'll ask you some routine questions first. Then he'll explain everything to you and make sure you feel completely comfortable.

Susan Great. Will he examine my breasts, too?

Meike Yes, he'll ask you to undress and he'll examine your breasts while you stand in front of him. He'll show you how to do a self-exam, too. Look, would you like me to be present?

Susan No, it's OK. I think I'll be all right.

Meike You will be, don't worry.

Susan What happens after that?

Meike Then you lie down on the exam table. He has to take what we call a smear test – which is taking some cells from your cervix using a tiny wooden stick and a special brush. Don't worry, it's just routine, but it means we can send the cells for testing and make sure everything is absolutely as it should be.

Susan Is that everything?

Meike Almost. Last of all, the doctor does a quick internal examination to make sure all your internal organs are just as they should be. It won't hurt, but if you do feel any discomfort, tell the doctor right away. The doctor will explain in more detail exactly what he's going to do at each step of the examination. He's very gentle and really friendly, you know. Just sit down and relax, Susan. He'll be with you in a minute or two. OK?

Susan OK. Thanks.

Track 24: Unit 6, Exercise 16B

Good afternoon everyone. My name is Joyce Reynolds and I'm here today to talk to you about the relationship between a patient and a carer. The success of everything we do as carers relies on trust and human understanding.

Our patients' situation means that they need other people to do some of the basic and personal tasks for them. However, they still have the same human dignity as everyone else. So we must always, therefore, show warmth, understanding and respect. This means always remembering a few simple, but very important, points.

Firstly, as we all know, patients often get angry and frustrated. It's essential to keep calm, not react and not take it personally. Try to find out why the patient is angry. The patient might not even know that he or she is ill-tempered and even if they do, they might not know why. They are probably lonely or worried rather than angry with you.

Secondly, by doing too much for a patient you can create a feeling of helplessness and weakness. Even worse, the patient can become lazy and simply expect you to do everything, which will make your job harder and reduce their self-respect. So, remember to let the patients do things for themselves – it will make your life easier and increase their self-esteem.

Next, it's important to remember the job is all about people. But rushing around doing jobs for the patient can mean that there is little or no time to actually be with the patient. If the patient thinks you are too busy, he or she might not even try to talk to you. And remember: listening is one of the most important things a carer does.

Honesty is the next point. If the patient is angry because of something you have done, tell the truth, apologize and try to put things right. Don't make the same mistake again. Always tell the truth. If you have forgotten something, say so. Without honesty there can be no trust.

And finally, don't forget to take care of yourself, as well. As a carer, you get tired and frustrated. Take time off to relax and do things you enjoy. Make sure that there's someone you can talk to about the difficulties of the job. You could talk to your manager, but sometimes it is better to talk to someone outside of work.

Track 25: Unit 7, Exercise 3A

Narrator First caller.
Hotline Good morning, NHS Nutrition Hotline. How can I help you?
Caller 1 Oh, good morning. Could you give me some information about a healthy diet during pregnancy, please?
Hotline Certainly. One of the best things I can recommend for pregnant women is folic acid. You find it in fruit and vegetables such as cabbage, broccoli and spinach. It's also in high-fibre food such as bread and cereals.
Caller 1 What about vitamins? Should I take extra vitamins?
Hotline Well, some are more useful than others. Vitamin C and D, for example, are very good for you, but too much vitamin A or B can be dangerous. You should really discuss this with your doctor.
Caller 1 Oh, I see. Umm, I have another question. Is it really true that you can't drink any alcohol while you're pregnant?
Hotline Yes, you really shouldn't. Alcohol can harm the foetus. And don't forget: no smoking either.
Caller 1 It's OK, I'm not a smoker, anyway. Oh, one other thing …

Narrator Second caller.
Hotline Good morning, NHS Nutrition Hotline. How can I help you?
Caller 2 Hello. I have a question about the labels on some products. When I read them, I see there are lots of different types of oils and fats. Could you tell me what the difference is between them and which ones are healthier than others?
Hotline Well, first, there are vegetable oils, like olive oil and rapeseed oil, for example. And then there are animal fats.
Caller 2 By animal fats, you mean butter, right?
Hotline Yes, butter and fat found in other dairy products, like milk or yoghurt, but also fat from meat like beef, pork, chicken …
Caller 2 I see.
Hotline Some vegetable oils, like olive oil or rapeseed oil – in the USA this is called 'canola oil' – are a lot healthier for you than animal fats. Too much animal fat in your diet can cause high blood pressure and heart problems because they increase the cholesterol levels in the blood.
Caller 2 What are the most dangerous types of fats?
Hotline Well, beef fat is more harmful than fats found in chicken and fish. And some vegetable oils, like coconut oil or palm oil, are just as bad. They're all high in something called saturated fats. Doctors say we should limit the amount of saturated fats in our diets.
Caller 2 Err, what do you mean by the word 'saturated'?
Hotline Well, all the fat we eat …

Narrator Third caller.
Hotline Good morning, NHS Nutrition Hotline. How can I help you?
Caller 3 Good morning. I'm calling about baby food products.
Hotline OK. Any products in particular?
Caller 3 Yes, my baby daughter really likes drinking sweet tea, but a friend of mine said that it isn't good for her. Is that true?
Hotline Well, sweet tea contains a lot of sugar and too much sugar is very bad for your baby's teeth. So, yes, unsweetened teas are better for her.
Caller 3 But what if she doesn't like them? I think my daughter has a bit of a sweet tooth, so she might not like unsweetened tea.
Hotline Well, some fruit teas don't need any sugar because they are naturally sweet. In fact, some fruit teas are naturally sweeter than some of the teas sweetened with sugar. They are some of the most popular baby products. They're very good. But you can also buy some baby drinks that taste sweet but don't have any sugar in them. Maybe you can try the unsweetened fruit teas first and if your daughter really doesn't like them, then you could try the others.
Caller 3 OK, I'll do that. Thanks for your help. Bye.

Track 27: Unit 8, Exercise 1A

Woman Eating disorders are a growing problem for young people today. With glossy magazines full of size zero, it's easy to see why teenagers are suffering from low self-esteem and problems with accepting their weight. With me today is Dr Sanjay Sohail, who is an expert on eating disorders. Good morning, Dr Sohail.
Dr Sohail Good morning.
Woman First of all, what are the most common eating disorders?
Dr Sohail Well, there are three main disorders: anorexia, bulimia and overeating.
Woman And how are they different?
Dr Sohail Basically, anorexia is when someone doesn't eat enough to keep their body weight. Overeating is when someone eats far more than they need to keep their body weight, and bulimia is overeating followed by purging.
Woman What do you mean by 'purging'?
Dr Sohail Purging is when someone overeats and then makes themselves vomit to bring all the food back up in order to control their body weight.
Woman Now, parents often don't see the symptoms soon enough. So maybe you could tell us how to spot these illnesses.
Dr Sohail Well, people who suffer from anorexia and bulimia starve their body of the food and energy it needs, which can lead to serious weight loss. It can also lead to poor circulation, low blood pressure, feeling cold, headaches, and no energy or enthusiasm. Because the body also doesn't get the vitamins it needs, hair loss is common as is the growth of facial hair. Malnutrition also leads to dental problems. Bulimics eat large amounts of food because they are depressed, then

they purge by either vomiting it back up or using a strong laxative.

Woman It all sounds horrible! And what about overeating? We hear a lot about teenage obesity nowadays.

Dr Sohail Being overweight is the easiest symptom to see. Sufferers often have high blood pressure and a fast or irregular heart rate. All these illnesses can lead to depression, too, of course.

Woman And what can parents do when they see these symptoms?

Dr Sohail I think it's very important that they don't try to deal with it themselves. They should talk to their family doctor and …

Track 28: Unit 8, Exercise 3A and 3B

Presenter Hello, and welcome back. Now, I don't know about you but it seems to me that kids nowadays are getting bigger and bigger. There's lots of talk about teenagers eating junk food and playing video games all day, but I wonder, are kids really getting bigger? And if so, why? So, with me in the studio is Dr Sherry Bonheim from the National Obesity Forum. So, Sherry, are kids getting bigger?

Expert Yes, they are. A new study shows that amongst 10 to 17-year-olds, about 30 per cent of kids are now overweight or obese. In 49 US states, one in five people are now obese.

Presenter One in five! That's incredible. But how overweight is 'obese'?

Expert People with a BMI of over 30 are …

Presenter BM what?

Expert BMI. Body mass index. It's your weight in kilograms divided by the square of your height in metres. A healthy BMI is between 18 and 25, anything over 30 is obese.

Presenter But why are so many people overweight?

Expert Well, there are many reasons. There has been a lot of research and it seems kids today do far less physical activity than before. And kids are eating a lot more calories, too.

Presenter People are eating more …

Expert Yes, and less healthy food – more fast food and high-calorie foods.

Presenter And what else does research tell us?

Expert It also tells us that kids hang out with other kids of the same weight and copy each other's eating habits.

Presenter So fat friends can make you overweight!

Expert Yes, so it seems …

Presenter But what about parents? Surely they play a part in this?

Expert They do. If dad's overweight, then he's less likely to go out and play soccer with the kids, so they join him on the couch and watch TV together.

Presenter And how big a problem is all this?

Expert Well, obesity increases the risk of type 2 diabetes and there are now over 20 million Americans with diabetes. Health care spending on obesity rose by 37 per cent between 1996 and 2008 and now costs the US over 150 billion dollars a year.

Presenter Now, that's what I call a big problem! But what can we do about …

Track 29: Unit 9, Exercise 1A

Dr Schneider Good morning, Mrs Brady. How can I help you today?

Shelly Brady Good morning, Doctor. I was checking my breasts and I found what I think might be a lump.

Dr Schneider OK, first of all, self-examination is a very sensible thing to do, so that's good. When did you first notice something?

Shelly Brady It was a few days ago. I didn't want to make a big fuss but I've been very worried about it.

Dr Schneider No, no, you did the right thing. You should always get anything suspicious checked. Is it painful at all?

Shelly Brady Not really, only when I put a lot of pressure on it.

Dr Schneider And is it just one thing you found? Or more?

Shelly Brady Just one. I only found one. On my left breast.

Dr Schneider And do you know if there is any history of breast cancer in your family at all?

Shelly Brady No, I don't think so. Not that I know of.

Dr Schneider That's good to hear. When did you last have a mammogram?

Shelly Brady Oh, erm, maybe two years ago.

Dr Schneider And where are you in your cycle at the moment?

Shelly Brady My last period finished last week.

Dr Schneider OK, and one last question, are you breast-feeding at all at the moment?

Shelly Brady No, no. My children are all at school!

Dr Schneider Right, OK then, let's take a look and see if we can find anything.

Track 31: Unit 9, Exercise 4B

Dr Schneider OK, right. Are you comfortable, Mrs Brady?

Shelly Brady Yes, thanks.

Dr Schneider Good. Now, could you please put your left arm up and behind your head? That's it. Lovely, thank you. Is the pillow nice and comfortable?

Shelly Brady Yes, it's fine, thanks.

Dr Schneider OK. Now, I'm just going to put some special acoustic gel on your breast so the scanner gives me a better image. Don't worry, it's not going to mark your skin or clothing. But at first it may be a bit cold! (laughs) And now I'm going to press the scanner into the breast and have a look at what we have in there. Just a bit of gentle pressure, it won't hurt. Is that comfortable?

Shelly Brady Yes, that's fine.

Dr Schneider Good. That's it. Now, could I ask you to just turn onto your right side, please? So I can get a good image of the outside of the breast. That's it, thank you.

Shelly Brady Am I going to get the results of the scan today? I really am very worried that it might be cancer.

Dr Schneider Yes, sure, we'll discuss the results when we've finished. And there's no need to panic and no point in worrying until we have all the facts. Most lumps are simple cysts and are benign and not serious at all. And even if it is a malignant tumour, the recovery rates nowadays are very high. So, don't worry, Mrs Brady, you're in good hands. It's perfectly normal. OK, that's it. Thank you. Right, I'm going to let you clean the gel off and get dressed again and then we'll talk about the results.

Shelly Brady	OK, fine.
	...
Dr Schneider	Please sit down. Right, now there is something there inside the breast but, as I said, there is no need to panic. It's only small and it's not clear from the ultrasound whether it's malignant or not. So, what I'm going to do is refer you for an appointment with a specialist tomorrow for what we call a digital mammogram – then we will know for sure what is there and whether we need to take any action. This is all very routine, so don't worry. We don't know for sure yet if it is serious, but we will do tomorrow.

Track 32: Unit 9, Exercise 5A

Good morning, my name's Dr Sanders and today I'm going to talk to you about screening patients for alcohol problems. First we're going to look at when to screen and then how to do it, and finally, what to do when you think there is a problem with alcohol use. This'll take about 20 minutes and I'll give you some handouts at the end of the presentation.

So, Step 1 is When to screen. Screening can be part of any routine examination but should always be done when prescribing any medication that interacts with alcohol or when seeing patients who are pregnant or trying to get pregnant. High-risk patients such as smokers, adolescents and young adults should also be screened. Also patients with health problems that might be alcohol related, such as depression or liver disease.

Once you have decided to screen, then you go to the second step which is Prescreen. Now, what does that exactly mean?
Well, you simply ask the patient about their alcohol use. When? How often? How much? If they drink, then ask them to complete this questionnaire. I'll hand out a copy for you all at the end of my presentation. Now, if a patient's answers don't show heavy drinking, then remind them of the recommended limits, and that's the end of the screening. But if the questionnaire is positive, you move to Step 3 and assess for alcohol-use disorders.

The key question in this step concerns the patient's relationships. So, you need to ask about this. For example, is the patient having problems with relationships with family, with friends, with a partner or with colleagues at work? Those are the main areas. If they answer yes to one or two of these questions, then there are no serious problems and you simply remind them of the recommended limits, and that's the end of the screening.
If they answer yes to three or more of these, they are showing alcohol dependence, and we move to Step 4: Advise and Assist.

The first thing you need to do in this step is to tell the patient they have an alcohol-use disorder. You need to explain the risks to them. They often don't know or don't want to know about the risks. Then you need to say that your role is to work with them to reduce their alcohol consumption or help them stop drinking completely. In order to do this, agree a drinking goal with them. This is important. But even more important, make a follow-up appointment with the patient. And stress that this appointment must be kept.

This takes us to Step 5: Follow-up. Keep notes on how well the patient is meeting their agreed drinking goal. If they are, then continue support for at least three months.
If they aren't, then we move to the final step, Step 6: Referral to a specialist.

But before you refer the patient to a specialist, you should first recommend a support group such as Alcoholics Anonymous and then also talk about the possibility of prescribing medication. Change is difficult, tell the patient you understand that, but explain why it's so important for them to stop or reduce their drinking.

Track 33: Unit 10, Exercise 3

Ulrike, aged 24
Well, it's a bit harder for me because I'm not actually British. I'm living in England because my husband is British. We moved here two years ago and I've been working in shops and stuff. But I trained as a doctor's assistant in Germany, so I'd like to make use of my training and start a career in the UK. The trouble is, you don't really have a similar qualification in the UK and you don't have doctor's assistants here. When I worked in a small practice in Germany for three years, for example, I did all the reception work and helped the doctor treat patients. No one does both jobs in the UK. I'll need to learn what software is used here, but I'm sure that won't be a problem.

Sharon, aged 32
I worked as a general practice nurse for six years before I stopped to have children. Before I stopped, I was a team leader responsible for a team of five nurses. I'd got my RN qualification and was studying for a post-graduate diploma. One of my children is disabled, so I've learned a lot about caring for the disabled while I've been a full-time mother. I'd like to go back to full-time work now my children are at school.

Tom, aged 17
I'm about to finish school and I really want to find a job, but I haven't really got any qualifications. I'm doing a Saturday job at the moment in an old people's home, which I really enjoy. The old people have lots of really interesting stories about what life was like when they were young. Sometimes they're really funny, as well. I wouldn't mind working with old people as a full-time job if I could find one.

Kate, aged 22
When I left school, I went to college and did a course in Health and Social Care. I worked with old people for a while and really enjoyed it, but I lost my job after about a year. So, I went to a temping agency and did some temporary secretarial jobs for a while. I think I'm good at getting on with people and I'd like to work with the elderly again. What else? Well, I'm good with computers and I think I'm also pretty good at organizing.

Track 34: Unit 10, Exercise 12

Presenter	So, next we're going to talk about job interviews. With the help of my next guest, you too can go into a job interview feeling relaxed and confident. So, welcome Sophie McKenzie, from Elite Employment. Hello Sophie.
Sophie	Hi.
Presenter	So, Sophie. It's the day of the interview. What can you do to make it all less stressful?
Sophie	Well, the day of the interview is too late to start thinking about it. You need to do lots of preparation beforehand!
Presenter	Oh, right. And what kind of preparation is that?
Sophie	Well, for a start, find out everything you can about the company. Can you find information about them

on the internet, for example? Can you talk to someone who works there? And always make sure you know where the interview will be. How long will it take you to get there? If you're going by car, what will the traffic be like at that time of day? Never be late for an interview.

Presenter That all sounds very sensible. What else can you do to prepare?

Sophie Find out about the job. Read the advertisement very carefully, several times. If you need to, change your CV to match it the best you can and think carefully about how to explain why you are right for the job. Practise the interview with a friend. Record it and listen to how you sound. Don't forget, practice makes perfect.

Presenter And what about appearances? How important is it to look smart?

Sophie Very important. Always choose clothes that are smart but comfortable. Avoid lots of jewellery or clothes that look sexy. Don't wear new clothes or shoes for the first time as they may be uncomfortable. Once again, plan in advance.

Presenter OK, that's lots of preparation, but what about the big day itself?

Sophie The best preparation starts the evening before your interview. Have a relaxing bath. It will help you to relax and get a good night's sleep. Get up early enough so that you have enough time for a good healthy breakfast and give yourself plenty of time to get to the Interview.

Presenter That's great advice. Thank you very much Sophie McKenzie.

KMK Mock Exam: B1

REZEPTION I (Hörverstehen)

Christine I see from your menu that you do not only have dishes for vegetarians but also for people with different religious backgrounds. That's quite unusual, isn't it?

Doug That's right. Apart from serving a wide variety of international dishes and specialities, we also cater for various religions. Although there are quite a number of vegetarian restaurants here in town, there aren't many places offering special menus for international customers.

Christine I see. What problems do you face when preparing meals for Muslims and Hindus, for example?

Doug Well, let's take Muslims first. Food such as bacon, ham or any food containing pork in any form is forbidden for them. In addition, they are not allowed to eat crab, lobster or shrimps. Now, we are famous for our shellfish dishes, but unfortunately they cannot appear on the menu for Muslims. So, we have to avoid all these foods.

Christine Ah yes, this was a custom that evolved many years ago to avoid food poisoning in hot desert countries, wasn't it?

Doug Yes, that's true. But not only that. It's part of their faith and culture. After all, how many Christians would be happy to eat horse, cat or even mice?

Christine Hmm, I take the point. And what about Hindus? Is it the same for them?

Doug No. Hindus don't eat beef because cows are sacred. And obviously they don't eat veal, either. You know, the meat of young cows. So, that reduces the range of food we can offer them. And, unfortunately some of our superb veal dishes simply can't be on the menu. But the good news is that we have a large selection of special Indian dishes. The other point that affects us is that for some religions there are periods in the calendar with restrictions such as eating only vegetarian food. But this is not a problem for us – the guests just choose from our vegetarian menu.

Christine I see. Now, tell me, is it OK for you when you have guests asking you about what is in the dish, or what sort of meat it is or how it was cooked and all these sorts of questions?

Doug No, no, that's fine, we're happy to explain. This is their culture, they need to know, and we respect that. No problem. In principle, it's no different from, say, the Greek habit of someone coming straight into the kitchen to see what's on the menu. After all, we have nothing to hide!

Christine OK, I see. Now, tell me about 'kosher' food.

Doug I must admit Jewish catering is much more complicated, following as it does, the strict dietary laws and traditions laid down in the Jewish religion.

Christine So, what sort of problems do you have there?

Doug There's an extremely complex set of guidelines which include restrictions on how meat is slaughtered, which animals, birds or seafood may be eaten. As most people know, pork and shellfish are not allowed. Well, to cut a long story short, our chefs know how to prepare kosher food, and our customers from Israel can trust them. And do you know what? Many non-Jewish people prefer foods marked kosher because they believe them to be cleaner and more strictly prepared.

Christine Oh, I see.

Doug Oh, and before I forget, there is another prohibition which we need to watch: staff are not allowed to use equipment that has come into contact with milk for preparing meat either in the kitchen or in the food service area. After a meal of meat Jews are not permitted to drink milk for four hours.

Christine That's interesting. I didn't know that. Well, thank you very much, Doug, I've learnt a lot today – and especially about how difficult it must be to please every customer.

UP Useful phrases

Talking about numbers

Cardinal numbers		Ordinal numbers	
0	oh/nought/null (AE) zero		
1	one	1st	first
2	two	2nd	second
3	three	3rd	third
4	four	4th	fourth
5	five	5th	fifth
6	six	6th	sixth
7	seven	7th	seventh
8	eight	8th	eighth
9	nine	9th	ninth
10	ten	10th	tenth
11	eleven	11th	eleventh
12	twelve	12th	twelfth
13	thirteen	13th	thirteenth
14	fourteen	14th	fourteenth
15	fifteen	15th	fifteenth
16	sixteen	16th	sixteenth
17	seventeen	17th	seventeenth
18	eighteen	18th	eighteenth
19	nineteen	19th	nineteenth
20	twenty	20th	twentieth
21	twenty-one	21st	twenty-first
22	twenty-two	22nd	twenty-second
23	twenty-three	23rd	twenty-third
24	twenty-four	24th	twenty-fourth
30	thirty	30th	thirtieth
40	forty	40th	fortieth
50	fifty	50th	fiftieth
60	sixty	60th	sixtieth
70	seventy	70th	seventieth
80	eighty	80th	eightieth
90	ninety	90th	ninetieth
100	one hundred	100th	one hundredth

In English you say:

101	one hundred **and** one
235	two hundred **and** thirty-five
1,563,765 1 563 765	one million, five hundred **and** sixty-three thousand, seven hundred and sixty-five

You use commas or spaces (and not a point) after the thousands (or millions) in large numbers.

Decimals

In English, you write decimals with a point, not a comma.

0.25	oh/nought point two five (BE) zero point two five (AE)
3.76	three point seven six
55.37	fifty-five point three seven
1.585	one point five eight five

Fractions

¼	a/one quarter
⅓	a/one third
½	a/one half
⅔	two-thirds
¾	three-quarters
5/16	five sixteenths
1½	one and a half

1 m^2	one **square** metre		
1 m^3	one **cubic** metre		
5^2	five **squared**		
10^4	ten **to the power** of four		
+	plus	x	times/multiply by
–	minus	÷	divide by

Talking about measurements

Taking temperature

The 'normal' body temperature is 37 °C (thirty-seven degrees Centigrade/Celsius). That's 98.6 °F (ninety-eight point six degrees Fahrenheit).

- He has a temperature of 38 °C.
- She's ill in bed with a temperature of 102 °F.
- If your temperature goes above 100 °F, give me a call.

Measuring blood pressure (BP)

- Your blood pressure's normal. It's 120/80 (one twenty over eighty).
- He's suffering from high blood pressure. Today's reading is 185/100 (one eighty-five over one hundred).

Other measurements and their abbreviations

mg	milligram
g	gram
kg	kilogram
oz	ounce (= 28.35 g)
lb	pound (= 0.454 kg)
st	stone (= 6.356 kg)

ml	millilitre
cl	centilitre
l	litre
tsp	teaspoon
tbl	tablespoon

Conversion tables

Length:

1 inch	=	2.54 cm
1 foot	=	30.48 cm
1 yard	=	91.44 cm
1 mile	=	1.609 km
1 cm	=	0.3937 inches
1 m	=	39.37 inches
1 km	=	0.62137 miles

Area:

1 square inch (in^2)	=	6.45 cm^2
1 square foot (ft^2)	=	0.093 m^2
1 square mile (m^2)	=	2.59 km^2
1 cm^2	=	0.155 square inches
1 m^2	=	10.764 square feet
1 km^2	=	0.3861 square miles

Volume:

1 cubic inch (in^3)	=	16.387 cm^3
1 pint (pt.)	=	0.57 l
1 gallon (gal.)	=	4.546 l
1 US gallon	=	3.785 l
1 cm3	=	0.061 cubic inch
1 m^3	=	35.315 cubic feet
1 litre (l)	=	1.76 pints
1 litre (l)	=	0.22 gallons

Mass:

1 pound (lb)	=	0.453 kg
1 ton (t)	=	1016 kg
1 kilogram (kg)	=	2.2046 pounds

Temperature:

Degrees Celsius		Degrees Fahrenheit
−17.8 °C	=	0 °F
−12.2 °C	=	10 °F
−6.7 °C	=	20 °F
−1.1 °C	=	30 °F

You say: −5 °C minus five degrees Celsius
−25.5 °C minus twenty-five point five degrees Celsius

0 °C	=	32 °F
4.4 °C	=	40 °F
10 °C	=	50 °F
20 °C	=	68 °F
30 °C	=	86 °F
40 °C	=	104 °F
50 °C	=	122 °F

Absolute zero = −273.15 °C

Energy:

1 joule = 0.2388 calories (cal)

Talking about time and dates

Telling the time

7.00	7 o'clock (in the morning) seven a.m.
7.05	5 minutes past seven seven oh five a.m.
7.15	(a) quarter past seven seven fifteen a.m.
7.30	half past seven seven thirty a.m.
7.45	(a) quarter to eight seven forty-five a.m.
7.57	3 minutes to/before eight seven fifty-seven a.m.
12.00	twelve o'clock (noon/midday)
3.00	three o'clock (in the afternoon) three p.m.
3.30	half past three three thirty p.m.
12.00	twelve o'clock (at night) midnight

a.m. = from 0.00 to 12.00 (you say: ay – em)
p.m. = from 12.00 to 0.00 (you say: pee – em)
o'clock is only used for the full hour

Formal:
What time is it, please?
Can you tell me what the time is, please?
Informal:
What's the time?

What's the date today?

you write:	you say:
8 July	It's the eighth of July.
8th August	It's the eighth of August
July 8th	It's July the eighth. (BE) It's July eighth. (AE)

Be careful:
8.7.17 means '8 July 2017' in the UK, but 'August 7, 2017' in the USA!

Days of the week

Monday (Mon), Tuesday (Tues), Wednesday (Wed), Thursday (Thurs), Friday (Fri), Saturday (Sat), Sunday (Sun)

B Basic word list

Diese Liste enhält ca. 500 Grundwörter, die in *Health Matters 3rd edition* als bekannt vorausgesetzt werden. Nicht aufgeführt, jedoch vorausgesetzt sind einige elementare Wörter wie Pronomen, Zahlen, Wochentage und Monatsnamen (z. B. *she, ten, Monday, January* usw.).

A

able, be ~ fähig/in der Lage sein
about über, ungefähr
above über, oben, oberhalb
address Adresse
adult Erwachsene/r
after nach, nachdem
afternoon Nachmittag
again wieder
age Alter
all alle
already schon, bereits
also auch, außerdem
always immer
animal Tier
another noch eine/r/s, ein/e andere/r/s
answer Antwort; beantworten
any irgendetwas, irgendwelche/r/s, jede/r/s
anybody jemand, jeder
anyone jemand, jede/r
anywhere irgendwo, irgendwohin
apple Apfel
area Gegend, Umgebung, Gebiet, Bereich
arm Arm
around herum, ungefähr
arrive ankommen, eintreffen
as wie, als
ask fragen, bitten

B

back zurück
bad schlecht, schlimm
bag Tüte, Tasche
bank Bank, Ufer
basic grundlegend, wesentlich, einfach
be sein
because da, weil
become werden
bed Bett
beer Bier
before vor, vorher
begin anfangen, beginnen
beginning Anfang
between zwischen
big groß, dick
biology Biologie
birthday Geburtstag
bit, a ~ ein bisschen
black schwarz
blue blau
body Körper
book Buch, Heft
boss Chef/in
both beide
bottle Flasche
box Kasten, Kiste, Schachtel
boy Junge
bread Brot
breakfast Frühstück
bring (mit)bringen, holen
Britain Großbritannien
British Brite/Britin; britisch
bus stop Bushaltestelle
business Handel, Gewerbe, Geschäft, Unternehmen
butter Butter
buy kaufen

C

cake Kuchen
called, be ~ heißen
can dürfen, können
car Auto
card Karte
cash Bargeld
central zentral
certainly sicherlich, natürlich
chair Stuhl
cheese Käse
child, children Kind, Kinder
chocolate Schokolade, Praline
cigarette Zigarette
cinema Kino
city (Groß-)Stadt
class Klasse
clean sauber; reinigen, säubern
climb klettern, steigen
clock Uhr
close schließen
coffee Kaffee
cold kalt
colour Farbe
come kommen
contact Kontakt
control Kontrolle; kontrollieren, überwachen, steuern
correct richtig, korrekt; berichtigen, korrigieren
cost Kosten; kosten
could konnte/n, könnte/n
count zählen
country Land, Staat
course, of ~ natürlich, selbstverständlich
cup Tasse
cut schneiden

D

danger Gefahr
dangerous(ly) gefährlich
dark dunkel
date Datum
daughter Tochter
day Tag
dead tot
dear liebe/r
deep(ly) tief
department store Warenhaus
desk Schreibtisch
dialogue Dialog, Gespräch
dictionary Wörterbuch
difficult schwierig
direct(ly) direkt
discuss diskutieren, erörtern
do tun, machen
doctor Doktor, Arzt/Ärztin
door Tür
down (nach) unten, herunter
dream Traum; träumen
drink Getränk; trinken
drive fahren
dry trocknen; trocken
during während

E

each jede/r/s, jeweils
each other einander, gegenseitig
early früh
earring Ohrring
easy einfach, leicht
eat essen
e.g. z.B.
egg Ei
end Ende
energy Energie
evening Abend
ever je(mals), schon (ein)mal
every jede/r/s
everybody jede/r
everything alles
exact(ly) exakt, genau
exam Prüfung
example Beispiel

example, for ~ zum Beispiel
explain erklären, erläutern
excuse me Entschuldigung
exercise Übung
exercise book (Schul-)Heft
expensive teuer

F
fact Tatsache
fall fallen, stürzen
false falsch
family Familie
far weit (entfernt); weitaus
fashion Mode
fast schnell
fat Fett; dick, fett
favourite Lieblings-
feel (sich) fühlen, der Meinung sein
finally schließlich, zum Schluss
find finden, suchen
fine gut, in Ordnung
finish (be)enden, aufhören (mit)
finished fertig
first erste/r/s, zuerst, zunächst
fish Fisch(e)
food Essen, Nahrung, Lebensmittel
foot, feet Fuß, Füße
football Fußball
forget vergessen
form Form, Formular
free kostenlos, frei
friend Freund/in
friendly freundlich
front, in ~ of vor
fruit Obst, Frucht, Früchte
full voll, vollständig
fun Spaß
funny lustig, komisch
future Zukunft

G
game Spiel
geography Geographie
German Deutsche/r; deutsch; Deutsch
Germany Deutschland
get bekommen, werden, gelangen
girl Mädchen
give geben
glass Glas
glasses Brille
go gehen, fahren
good gut
goodbye auf Wiedersehen
grammar Grammatik
great groß; toll, prima
green grün
group Gruppe

H
hair Haar/e
half Hälfte; halb
happy froh, zufrieden, glücklich
hard schwierig, hart
have haben
head Kopf
health Gesundheit
hear hören
heavy schwer
help Hilfe; helfen
here hier
high hoch
hold halten, festhalten
holiday Ferien, Urlaub
home Zuhause, Heim
hope Hoffnung; hoffen
hospital Krankenhaus
hot heiß, warm
hour Stunde
how wie
however jedoch, allerdings
hunger Hunger
hungry hungrig
husband Ehemann

I
ice Eis
idea Idee, Gedanke, Vorstellung
ideal genau richtig, ideal
ill krank
important wichtig
information Angaben, Information(en)
interest Interesse; interessieren
interesting interessant
into in ... hinein
Ireland Irland
Irish Ire/Irin, irisch

J
job Arbeit, Stelle

K
keep halten, behalten
key Schlüssel
kill töten
kitchen Küche
know kennen, wissen

L
language Sprache
large groß
last letzte/r/s; zuletzt
late spät, zu spät
learn lernen, erfahren
leave abfahren, verlassen
left links
leg Bein
less weniger
let lassen, zulassen
letter Brief, Buchstabe
level Niveau, Maß, Ebene, Spiegel, Wert(e)
life, lives Leben
like mögen, gern haben
line Linie, Zeile, Leitung
list Liste
listen anhören, zuhören
litre Liter
little klein, wenig
live wohnen, leben
long lang
look sehen, aussehen
look for suchen
lot, a ~ viel, viele
lots of viel, viele
love Liebe; lieben, sehr gern mögen
low niedrig, tief
lunch Mittagessen

M
machine Gerät
magazine Zeitschrift
make machen
man, men Mann, Männer
many viele
married (to) verheiratet (mit)
maths Mathe(matik) *(Schulfach)*
may dürfen, können
medium mittlere/r/s, mittel
meet treffen, kennen lernen
metal Metall
method Verfahren, Arbeitsweise
metre Meter
middle Mitte, mittlerer Teil
milk Milch
mineral water Mineralwasser
minute Minute
mistake Fehler
money Geld
month Monat
more mehr, weitere/r/s
morning Morgen, Vormittag
most am meisten
mother Mutter
mouth Mund
move bewegen
much viel
music Musik
must müssen

N
near nahe
nearly fast

necessary nötig, notwendig
need brauchen, benötigen
negative verneinend
never nie(mals)
new neu
newspaper Zeitung
next nächste/r/s, danach
next to neben
nice nett, schön
night Nacht
normal(ly) normal
nose Nase
nothing nichts
noun Nomen, Substantiv
now nun, jetzt
number Nummer, Zahl

O
o'clock ... Uhr
office Büro
often oft, häufig
old alt
onto auf
only nur; einzige/r/s
open öffnen; offen
opposite gegenüber
original original
other andere/r/s
over (vor)über, darüber

P
pair Paar
paper Papier, Zeitung
parents Eltern
park Park; parken
parking Parkmöglichkeiten, Parkplätze
part Teil
partner Partner/in
pay zahlen, bezahlen
pen Stift
people Menschen, Leute
perfect perfekt
person Mensch, Person
phone Telefon; anrufen
photo(graphy) Foto(grafie)
phrase Redewendung, Ausdruck
picture Bild
piece Stück
place Ort, Platz
plan Plan, Lageplan; planen
plane Flugzeug
please bitte
point Punkt
popular beliebt
possible möglich
post office Postamt
potato Kartoffel
pound Pfund (Sterling)
present Gegenwart; Geschenk
pretty hübsch
price (Kauf-)Preis
product Produkt, Erzeugnis
put setzen, stellen, legen

Q
question Frage
quick(ly) schnell
quiet leise, ruhig

R
rain Regen; regnen
read lesen
ready bereit, fertig
really wirklich, eigentlich
red rot
regular(ly) regelmäßig
rest Rest
right rechts, richtig
right, be ~ Recht haben
road Straße
role Rolle
room Zimmer, Raum
run laufen

S
safe sicher
salad Salat
salt Salz
same gleiche/r/s, der-, die-, dasselbe
say sagen
school Schule
second zweite/r/s
see sehen
sell verkaufen
send senden, (ver)schicken
sentence Satz
several einige, mehrere
shall sollen, werden
shirt Hemd
short kurz
should solle/n, sollte/n
show zeigen
side Seite
sign Zeichen, Anzeichen
silver Silber
sit sitzen
situation Lage, Situation
sleep schlafen
slow(ly) langsam
small klein
smoke rauchen
so also, damit
soft weich
some einige, etwas
somebody, someone jemand
something etwas
sometimes manchmal
somewhere irgendwo, irgendwohin
son Sohn
sorry Verzeihung. Tut mir Leid.
speak sprechen, reden
sport Sport
start anfangen
stay bleiben
still (immer) noch
stop anhalten, aufhören
story Geschichte
street Straße
strong stark
student Schüler/in, Student/in
sugar Zucker
summer Sommer
sweet Bonbon; süß

T
table Tisch, Tabelle
take nehmen, dauern
talk Gespräch; reden
tea Tee
telephone Telefon; anrufen
television (TV) Fernsehen
tell sagen, erzählen
test Untersuchung
thank danken
thank you danke
thanks Dank; danke
theatre Theater
then dann
there da, dort, dorthin
these diese
thing Sache, Ding
think denken, meinen, glauben, finden
those jene
through durch, hindurch
time Zeit; Mal
today heute
tomorrow morgen
tonight heute Abend/Nacht
top oberer Teil, oberste/r/s
tourist Tourist/in
town Stadt
toy Spielzeug
train Zug, Bahn
translate übersetzen
travel reisen
true wahr
type Art, Typ

U
under unter
understand verstehen

unhappy unglücklich
United Kingdom (UK) Vereinigtes Königreich
use Benutzung, Gebrauch; benutzen, gebrauchen
useful nützlich

V

vegetables Gemüse
verb Verb
very sehr
village Dorf
visit Besuch; besuchen
visitor Besucher/in
voice Stimme

W

wait warten
walk Spaziergang, Fußweg; (zu Fuß) gehen
wall Wand
want wollen
wash (sich) waschen
watch sehen, zusehen
watch TV fernsehen
water Wasser
way Weg, Art (und Weise)
weak schwach
wear *(Kleidung usw.)* tragen
week Woche
weekday Wochentag
weekend Wochenende
well gut; also
what was, welche/r/s
when wenn, als, wann
where wo, wohin
which welche/r/s
wish Wunsch; wünschen, wollen
white weiß
who wer, der/die/das
why warum
wife (Ehe-)Frau
will werde(n)
window Fenster
wine Wein
wish wünschen
with mit, bei
without ohne
woman, women Frau, Frauen
word Wort
work Arbeit; arbeiten
world Welt
would würde, würdest, würden
write schreiben
wrong falsch
wrong, be ~ Unrecht haben

Y

year Jahr
yellow gelb
yesterday gestern
young, younger jung, jünger

C Unit word list

In dieser Liste sind alle neuen Wörter – unter Voraussetzung des Grundwortschatzes (siehe *Basic word list*) – in der Reihenfolge ihres Vorkommens im Text verzeichnet. Es fehlen allerdings die Wörter der Abschnitte *KMK Exam Practice* der Units 1–10; diese Wörter werden als optional behandelt, sind aber im Alphabetischen Wörterverzeichnis (siehe *A–Z word list*) aufgeführt.
Die Zahl am Rand gibt die Seitenzahl an. T = Das Wort befindet sich im Transkript der Hörverständnistexte.

UNIT 1

6	**workplace** [ˈwɜːkpleɪs]	Arbeitsplatz
	typical [ˈtɪpɪkl]	typisch
	assistant [əˈsɪstənt]	Assistent/in, Helfer/in
	medical assistant [ˌmedɪkl əˈsɪstənt]	Medizinische Fachangestellte/r
	duty [ˈdjuːti]	Aufgabe
	to **match** [mætʃ]	zuordnen
	to **assist sb** [əˈsɪst]	jdm assistieren
	records *pl* [ˈrekɔːdz]	Akte(n), Unterlagen
	patient records *pl* [ˈpeɪʃnt rekɔːdz]	Patientenakte(n), Patientenunterlagen
	to **keep records** [ˌkiːp ˈrekɔːdz]	Akten halten, Unterlagen führen
	patient [ˈpeɪʃnt]	Patient/in
	to **look after sb** [lʊk ˈɑːftə]	sich um jdn kümmern
	appointment [əˈpɔɪntmənt]	Termin
	to **prepare** [prɪˈpeə]	(sich) vorbereiten
	surgical [ˈsɜːdʒɪkl]	chirurgisch
	surgical instruments *pl* [ˌsɜːdʒɪkl ˈɪnstrəmənts]	Operationsbesteck, chirurgische Instrumente
	equipment [ɪˈkwɪpmənt]	Ausstattung, Geräte
	blood [blʌd]	Blut
	blood sample [ˈblʌd sɑːmpl]	Blutprobe
7	to **describe** [dɪˈskraɪb]	beschreiben
	daily [ˈdeɪli]	täglich
	following [ˈfɒləʊɪŋ]	folgende/r/s
	care [keə]	Betreuung, Pflege
	to **organise** [ˈɔːgənaɪz]	organisieren
	surgery *BE* [ˈsɜːdʒəri]	(Arzt-)Praxis
	doctor's office *AE* [ˌdɒktəz ˈɒfɪs]	(Arzt-)Praxis
	lab(oratory) [læb, ləˈbɒrətri]	Labor
	administration [ədˌmɪnɪˈstreɪʃn]	Verwaltung
	statement [ˈsteɪtmənt]	Aussage, Schilderung
	to **make sure** [ˌmeɪk ˈʃʊə]	dafür sorgen
	to **treat** [triːt]	behandeln
	sterile [ˈsteraɪl]	steril
	front desk [ˌfrʌnt ˈdesk]	Rezeption, Anmeldung
	health centre [ˈhelθ sentə]	Gesundheitszentrum
	professional [prəˈfeʃənl]	professionell
	comfortable(-ably) [ˈkʌmftəbl]	angenehm, behaglich
	tidy [ˈtaɪdi]	ordentlich
	anxious [ˈæŋkʃəs]	ängstlich, besorgt, nervös
	upset [ˌʌpˈset]	aufgebracht, verstört
	to **try** [traɪ]	versuchen
	calm [kɑːm]	ruhig
	to **make sb do sth** [ˌmeɪk ˈduː]	jdn dazu bringen, etw zu tun
	to **relax** [rɪˈlæks]	sich entspannen
	to **enjoy doing sth** [ɪnˈdʒɔɪ]	etw gern tun
	boring [ˈbɔːrɪŋ]	langweilig
	to **analyse** [ˈænəlaɪz]	untersuchen, analysieren
	careful(ly) [ˈkeəfl]	sorgfältig, genau
	minor [ˈmaɪnə]	klein
	operation [ˌɒpəˈreɪʃn]	Operation
	exciting [ɪkˈsaɪtɪŋ]	spannend, aufregend
	note [nəʊt]	Notiz
	to **take notes** [ˌteɪk ˈnəʊts]	(sich) Notizen machen
	relaxed [rɪˈlækst]	locker, entspannt
	to **spend** [spend]	*(Zeit)* verbringen
	paperwork [ˈpeɪpəwɜːk]	Büroarbeit, Schreibarbeit(en)
	to **do paperwork** [duː ˈpeɪpəwɜːk]	Papierkram erledigen
	invoice [ˈɪnvɔɪs]	Rechnung
	up to date [ˌʌp tə ˈdeɪt]	auf dem neuesten Stand, aktuell
	accounts *pl* [əˈkaʊnts]	Buchhaltung
	to **order** [ˈɔːdə]	bestellen, in Auftrag geben
	supplies *pl* [səˈplaɪz]	Bedarf, Artikel, Waren
	to **be responsible for sth** [bi rɪˈspɒnsəbl fə]	für etw verantwortlich sein, für etw zuständig sein
	professional [prəˈfeʃənl]	beruflich
	culture [ˈkʌltʃə]	Kultur
	health care [ˈhelθ keə]	Gesundheitswesen, medizinische Versorgung
	General Practitioner (GP) *BE* [ˌdʒenrəl prækˈtɪʃənə]	Allgemeinarzt/-ärztin
	to **register (with sb)** [ˈredʒɪstə]	(sich) (bei jdm) anmelden
	in order to [ɪn ˈɔːdə tə]	um … zu
	to **receive** [rɪˈsiːv]	erhalten, bekommen
	to **move house** [ˌmuːv ˈhaʊs]	umziehen
	physician *AE* [fɪˈzɪʃn]	Arzt/Ärztin
	Primary Care Physician (PCP) *AE* [ˌpraɪməri ˈkeə fɪzɪʃn]	Allgemeinarzt/-ärztin
	general [ˈdʒenrəl]	allgemein
	insurance [ɪnˈʃʊərəns]	Versicherung
	health insurance [ˈhelθ ɪnʃʊərəns]	Krankenversicherung
	medical [ˈmedɪkl]	medizinisch, ärztlich

	you may find [jə ˌmeɪ ˈfaɪnd]	es kann sein, es kann vorkommen
8	**expression** [ɪkˈspreʃn]	Ausdruck
	the odd one out [ði ˌɒd wʌn ˈaʊt]	*etwas, was nicht dazugehört*
	reason [ˈriːzn]	Grund, Begründung
	to **give a reason** [ˌɡɪv ə ˈriːzn]	etw begründen
	choice [tʃɔɪs]	Wahl, Auswahl
	to **complete** [kəmˈpliːt]	vervollständigen
	to **smile** [smaɪl]	lächeln
	waiting room [ˈweɪtɪŋ ruːm]	Wartezimmer
	to **check** [tʃek]	überprüfen
	details *pl* [ˈdiːteɪlz]	Angaben, Daten
	individual [ˌɪndɪˈvɪdʒuəl]	Individuum
9	**X-rays** *pl* [ˈeksreɪz]	Röntgenstrahlen
	to **take X-rays** [ˌteik ˈeksreɪz]	röntgen
	(medical) receptionist [rɪˈsepʃənɪst]	Sprechstundenhilfe
	to **greet** [ɡriːt]	begrüßen
	practice [ˈpræktɪs]	Übung, Training
	below [bɪˈləʊ]	unten(stehend)
	complete [kəmˈpliːt]	vollständig
	nurse [nɜːs]	Krankenschwester/-pfleger
	to **collect** [kəˈlekt]	(ein)sammeln, kassieren
	fee [fiː]	Honorar, Gebühr
	private patient [ˌpraɪvət ˈpeɪʃnt]	Privatpatient/in
	pressure [ˈpreʃə]	Druck
	excellent [ˈeksələnt]	ausgezeichnet, hervorragend
	skills *pl* [skɪlz]	Fertigkeiten, Fähigkeiten
	magazine [ˌmæɡəˈziːn]	Zeitschrift
	medical supplies *pl* [ˌmedɪkl səˈplaɪz]	Sanitätsartikel
	to **tidy** [ˈtaɪdi]	aufräumen
	practice [ˈpræktɪs]	Praxis
	to **diagnose** [ˈdaɪəɡnəʊz]	diagnostizieren
	not … any more [nɒt ˌeni ˈmɔː]	nicht mehr
	electronic [ˌɪlekˈtrɒnɪk]	elektronisch
	booking [ˈbʊkɪŋ]	Reservierung
	injection [ɪnˈdʒekʃn]	Injektion, Spritze
10	to **give directions** [ˌɡɪv dəˈrekʃnz]	den Weg beschreiben
	directions *pl* [dəˈrekʃnz]	Wegbeschreibung
	to **call** [kɔːl]	anrufen
	map [mæp]	Karte, Plan
	to **refer to sth** [rɪˈfɜː tə]	sich auf etw beziehen
	(train) station [ˈsteɪʃn]	Bahnhof
	underground [ˈʌndəɡraʊnd]	U-Bahn

T	**sure** [ʃʊə]	sicher, (na) klar
	not … yet [ˌnɒt ˈjet]	noch nicht
	close (to sth) [kləʊs]	nahe (bei etw)

	main [meɪn]	Haupt-
	called [kɔːld]	namens
	straight on [ˌstreɪt ˈɒn]	geradeaus
	to **turn left/right** [tɜːn ˈleft, tɜːn ˈraɪt]	links/rechts abbiegen
	corner [ˈkɔːnə]	Ecke
	underground station [ˈʌndəɡraʊnd steɪʃn]	U-Bahn-Station
	northern [ˈnɔːðən]	nördlich, Nord-
	roundabout [ˈraʊndəbaʊt]	Kreisverkehr
	south [saʊθ]	Süden
	heading south [ˌhedɪŋ ˈsaʊθ]	in Richtung Süden
	north [nɔːθ]	Norden
	I'm afraid [aɪm əˈfreɪd]	leider
	parking spot [ˈpɑːkɪŋ spɒt]	Parkplatz

	to **draw** [drɔː]	zeichnen
	to **mark** [mɑːk]	markieren, kennzeichnen
	opposite [ˈɒpəzɪt]	gegenüber
12	**training** [ˈtreɪnɪŋ]	Ausbildung
	to **note** [nəʊt]	notieren, aufschreiben
	qualification [ˌkwɒlɪfɪˈkeɪʃn]	Abschluss, Qualifikation, Voraussetzung
	reception [rɪˈsepʃn]	Empfang, Rezeption
	intermediate [ˌɪntəˈmiːdiət]	mittel, Zwischen-
	diploma [dɪˈpləʊmə]	Diplom
	association [əˌsəʊsiˈeɪʃn]	Verband, Vereinigung
	medical secretary [ˌmedɪkl ˈsekrətri]	Arzthelfer/in (für Organisationsaufgaben)
	practice manager [ˌpræktɪs ˈmænɪdʒə]	Praxismanager/in
	medical administrator [ˌmedɪkl ədˈmɪnɪstreɪtə]	Arzthelfer/in (für Verwaltungsaufgaben)
	caring [ˈkeərɪŋ]	sozial (eingestellt)
	role [rəʊl]	Rolle
	within [wɪˈðɪn]	in, innerhalb
	environment [ɪnˈvaɪrənmənt]	Umfeld
	front line [ˌfrʌnt ˈlaɪn]	an vorderster Front
	staff [stɑːf]	Personal, Mitarbeiter/innen
	relative [ˈrelətɪv]	Verwandte/r
	either … or [ˌaɪðə(r) ˈɔː]	entweder … oder
	in person [ɪn ˈpɜːsn]	persönlich
	to **be involved in sth** [bi ɪnˈvɒlvd ɪn]	an etw beteiligt sein, mit etw zu tun haben
	to **choose** [tʃuːz]	wählen, auswählen
	to **book** [bʊk]	reservieren, buchen
	scheme [skiːm]	Programm, Projekt
	impression [ɪmˈpreʃn]	Eindruck
	to **affect** [əˈfekt]	beeinflussen
	opinion [əˈpɪniən]	Meinung, Ansicht
	organization [ˌɔːɡənaɪˈzeɪʃn]	Organisation, Unternehmen, Verband
	general practice [ˌdʒenrəl ˈpræktɪs]	Allgemeinarztpraxis
	clinic [ˈklɪnɪk]	Klinik

	to study for sth ['stʌdi fə]	sich auf etw vorbereiten, für etw lernen
	knowledge ['nɒlɪdʒ]	Wissen, Kenntnisse
	required [rɪ'kwaɪəd]	erforderlich, nötig
	challenging ['tʃælɪndʒɪŋ]	fordernd, anspruchsvoll
	to achieve [ə'tʃi:v]	erreichen, erlangen
	to gain a pass [ˌgeɪn ə 'pɑ:s]	eine Prüfung bestehen
	written ['rɪtn]	schriftlich
	examination/exam [ɪgˌzæmɪ'neɪʃn, ɪg'zæm]	Prüfung
	nationally set [ˌnæʃnəli 'set]	landesweit einheitlich
	assignment [ə'saɪnmənt]	Aufgabe
	to satisfy requirements [ˌsætɪsfaɪ rɪ'kwaɪəmənts]	Bedingungen erfüllen
	work experience ['wɜ:k ɪkspɪəriəns]	Berufs-/Arbeitserfahrung
	to pass [pɑ:s]	*(Prüfung)* bestehen
	work-based assignment [ˌwɜ:k beɪst ə'saɪnmənt]	praktische Prüfungsaufgabe
	programme *BE* ['prəʊgræm]	Programm
	available [ə'veɪləbl]	verfügbar, erhältlich
	full-time [ˌfʊl 'taɪm]	Vollzeit-
	part-time [ˌpɑ:t'taɪm]	Teilzeit-
	study ['stʌdi]	Studium, Ausbildung
	average ['ævərɪdʒ]	Durchschnitt, Durchschnitts-
	length [leŋθ]	Länge
	course [kɔ:s]	Kurs, Studiengang
	suitable ['su:təbl]	geeignet, passend
	both … and [bəʊθ ənd]	sowohl … als auch
	school leaver ['sku:l li:və]	Schulabgänger/in
	mature [mə'tʃʊə]	*hier:* älter/e
	member ['membə]	Mitglied
13	**feeling** ['fi:lɪŋ]	Gefühl, Ansicht, Meinung
	medical office *AE* [ˌmedɪkl 'ɒfɪs]	(Arzt-)Praxis
	certificate [sə'tɪfɪkət]	Urkunde, Zertifikat, Abschluss(zeugnis)
	program *AE* ['prəʊgræm]	Programm
	to cover ['kʌvə]	(ab)decken, *(Thema)* behandeln
	aspect ['æspekt]	Gesichtspunkt, Seite, Aspekt
	to perform sth [pə'fɔ:m]	etw ausüben
	key [ki:]	wichtigste/r/s, ausschlaggebend
	typically ['tɪpɪkli]	normalerweise, üblicherweise
	in the field [ɪn ðə 'fi:ld]	in der Praxis
	including [ɪn'klu:dɪŋ]	einschließlich
	documentation [ˌdɒkjumen'teɪʃn]	Unterlagen, Dokumentation
	scheduling ['ʃedju:lɪŋ]	Terminplanung
	to require sb to do sth [rɪ'kwaɪə]	von jdm verlangen, etw zu tun
	applicant ['æplɪkənt]	Bewerber/in
	certain ['sɜ:tn]	bestimmte/r/s
	experience [ɪk'spɪəriəns]	Erfahrung
	education [ˌedʒu'keɪʃn]	Schulbildung, Bildung
	class [klɑ:s]	Unterricht, Kurs
	common ['kɒmən]	üblich, gewöhnlich, verbreitet
	topic ['tɒpɪk]	Thema
	law [lɔ:]	Recht, Gesetz(e)
	ethics ['eθɪks]	Ethik
	delivery [dɪ'lɪvəri]	Umsetzung, Anwendung
	accounting [ə'kaʊntɪŋ]	Buchführung
	communication [kəˌmju:nɪ'keɪʃn]	Kommunikation
	degree [dɪ'gri:]	Abschluss
	associate degree *AE* [əˌsəʊʃiət dɪ'gri:]	*US-Abschluss, der nach zwei Jahren verliehen wird*
	coursework ['kɔ:swɜ:k]	Studieninhalt, Studienumfang
	successful(ly) [sək'sesfl]	erfolgreich
	to complete sth [kəm'pli:t]	etw abschließen, etw absolvieren
	to be equipped with sth [bi ɪ'kwɪpt wɪð]	mit etw ausgestattet sein, über etw verfügen
	anatomy [ə'nætəmi]	Anatomie
	first aid [ˌfɜ:st 'eɪd]	Erste Hilfe
	correspondence [ˌkɒrɪ'spɒndəns]	Schriftverkehr, Korrespondenz
	in addition to sth [ɪn ə'dɪʃn tə]	zusätzlich zu etw
	instruction [ɪn'strʌkʃn]	Unterricht
	on-site [ˌɒn 'saɪt]	vor Ort
	to supervise ['su:pəvaɪz]	beaufsichtigen, überwachen
	internship ['ɪntɜ:nʃɪp]	Praktikum
	to include [ɪn'klu:d]	einschließen, beinhalten
	clinical ['klɪnɪkl]	klinisch
	to assist [ə'sɪst]	helfen, unterstützen
	clinical assisting *AE* [ˌklɪnɪkl ə'sɪstɪŋ]	Behandlungsassistenz
	emergency [ɪ'mɜ:dʒənsi]	Notfall
	procedure [prə'si:dʒə]	Vorgehen, Verfahren(sweise)
	setting ['setɪŋ]	Rahmen, Umgebung
	process ['prəʊses]	Ablauf, Verfahren, Prozess
	usually ['ju:ʒuəli]	normalerweise, gewöhnlich
	to take place [ˌteɪk 'pleɪs]	stattfinden
	difference ['dɪfrəns]	Unterschied
	to employ sb [ɪm'plɔɪ]	jdn einstellen, jdn beschäftigen

UNIT 2

14	**urgent** ['ɜ:dʒənt]	dringend
	to have/take a look [həv/teɪk ə 'lʊk]	nachsehen, sich etw ansehen
	to fit sb in [ˌfɪt 'ɪn]	*(Termin:)* jdn einschieben, jdn dazwischenschieben
	to mean [mi:n]	bedeuten, heißen
	You're welcome. [jɔ: 'welkəm]	Bitte. Gern geschehen.

	treatment ['triːtmənt]	Behandlung
	due to ['djuː tə]	aufgrund von
	accident ['æksɪdənt]	Unfall
	illness ['ɪlnəs]	Krankheit
	European Economic Area [jʊərəˌpiːən iːkəˌnɒmɪk 'eəriə]	Europäischer Wirtschaftsraum
	to **entitle sb to sth** [ɪn'taɪtl]	jdm einen Anspruch auf etw verleihen
	state-provided ['steɪt prəvaɪdɪd]	staatlich
	politeness [pə'laɪtnəs]	Höflichkeit
	to **inconvenience sb** [ˌɪnkən'viːniəns]	jdm Unannehmlichkeiten bereiten
	response [rɪ'spɒns]	Reaktion, Antwort
15	to **make (it)** [meɪk]	(es) schaffen
T	**particular** [pə'tɪkjələ]	spezielle/r/s
	to **prefer** [prɪ'fɜː]	vorziehen, (lieber) mögen
	to **be busy** [bi 'bɪzi]	viel zu tun haben
	appointment book [ə'pɔɪntmənt bʊk]	Terminkalender
16	**pain** [peɪn]	Schmerz(en)
	to **be in pain** [bi ˌɪn 'peɪn]	Schmerzen haben
	prescription [prɪ'skrɪpʃn]	(ärztliches) Rezept, Verordnung
	result [rɪ'zʌlt]	Ergebnis, Resultat
	blood test ['blʌd test]	Blutuntersuchung
	spell [spel]	buchstabieren
	foreign ['fɒrən]	ausländisch, aus dem Ausland
	spelling ['spelɪŋ]	Schreibweise
T	to **take a seat** [ˌteɪk ə 'siːt]	Platz nehmen
17	**etiquette** ['etɪket]	Anstandsregel, Etikette
	to **deal with sb** ['diːl wɪð]	mit jdm umgehen, gegenüber jdm auftreten
	caller ['kɔːlə]	Anrufer/in
	image ['ɪmɪdʒ]	Bild (in der Öffentlichkeit), Image
	step [step]	Schritt
	to **allow** [ə'laʊ]	gestatten, erlauben
	to **call sb back** [ˌkɔːl 'bæk]	jdn zurückrufen
	case [keɪs]	Fall
	in case [ɪn 'keɪs]	für den Fall, dass; falls
	to **get disconnected** [get ˌdɪskə'nektɪd]	*(Telefonverbindung:)* unterbrochen werden
	courtesy ['kɜːtəsi]	Höflichkeit
	especially [ɪ'speʃəli]	besonders
	to **be happy to do sth** [bi 'hæpi tə duː]	etw gern tun
	prompt(ly) [prɒmpt]	unverzüglich, prompt
	to **confirm** [kən'fɜːm]	bestätigen
	ring [rɪŋ]	Klingeln
	clear(ly) [klɪə]	deutlich
	to **identify** [aɪ'dentɪfaɪ]	identifizieren, genau bestimmen
	to **provide** [prə'vaɪd]	bieten, liefern, zur Verfügung stellen
	service ['sɜːvɪs]	Dienstleistung, Service, Dienst
	to **deal with sth** ['diːl wɪð]	mit etw umgehen, etw erledigen, etw bearbeiten
	call [kɔːl]	(Telefon-)Anruf
	to **save (sb sth)** [seɪv]	(jdm etw) sparen
	to **put sb on hold** [ˌpʊt ɒn 'həʊld]	*(Telefon:)* jdn in die Warteschleife stellen
	permission [pə'mɪʃn]	Erlaubnis
	message ['mesɪdʒ]	Mitteilung, Nachricht
	to **take a message** [ˌteɪk ə 'mesɪdʒ]	*(Telefon:)* etw ausrichten
	urgency ['ɜːdʒənsi]	Dringlichkeit
	to **offer** ['ɒfə]	anbieten
	further ['fɜːðə]	weitere/r/s
	assistance [ə'sɪstəns]	Hilfe, Unterstützung
	by name [baɪ 'neɪm]	namentlich
	respect [rɪ'spekt]	Achtung, Respekt
	to **practise** ['præktɪs]	üben
18	**Australian** [ɒ'streɪliən]	Australier/in; australisch
	postcode ['pəʊstkəʊd]	Postleitzahl
	to **complete** [kəm'pliːt]	*(Formular usw.)* ausfüllen
	medical history [ˌmedɪkl 'hɪstri]	Krankengeschichte
	birth [bɜːθ]	Geburt
	first name ['fɜːst neɪm]	Vorname
	in general [ɪn 'dʒenrəl]	im Allgmeinen
	even ['iːvn]	sogar
	formal ['fɔːml]	formal, förmlich, formell
	colleague ['kɒliːg]	Kollege/-in
	customer ['kʌstəmə]	Kunde/-in
	normally ['nɔːməli]	normalerweise
	polite [pə'laɪt]	höflich
	title ['taɪtl]	Titel, Anrede
	surname ['sɜːneɪm]	Nachname
	date of birth [ˌdeɪt əv 'bɜːθ]	Geburtsdatum
19	**(patient) record file** ['rekɔːd faɪl]	Patientenakte, Patientendaten
	to **key in** [ˌkiː 'ɪn]	eintippen, *(Daten)* eingeben
	to **copy** ['kɒpi]	abschreiben
	missing ['mɪsɪŋ]	fehlend
	to **walk into sth** [ˌwɔːk 'ɪntə]	in etw (herein)kommen
	to **role-play** ['rəʊl pleɪ]	mit verteilten Rollen spielen
21	to **consider** [kən'sɪdə]	betrachten, in Betracht ziehen
	local ['ləʊkl]	ortsansässig, örtlich
	pharmacist ['fɑːməsɪst]	Apotheker/in
	outside [ˌaʊt'saɪd]	außerhalb
	hours *pl* ['aʊəz]	Öffnungszeiten, Sprechzeiten
	to **direct sb to sth** [də'rekt]	jdn auf etw verweisen, jdn umleiten

	out of hours [ˌaʊt əv ˈaʊəz]	außerhalb der Geschäfts-/ Sprechzeiten
	alternative(ly) [ɔ:lˈtɜ:nətɪv]	alternativ
	National Health Service (NHS) [ˌnæʃnəl ˈhelθ sɜ:vɪs]	Staatlicher Gesundheitsdienst
	advice [ədˈvaɪs]	Beratung, Rat
	life-threatening [ˈlaɪf θretnɪŋ]	lebensbedrohlich
	routine [ru:ˈti:n]	(Routine-)Vorgang, Verfahren
	professional [prəˈfeʃənl]	Fachmann/-frau
	to **enable** [ɪˈneɪbl]	ermöglichen, befähigen
	to **cancel** [ˈkænsl]	absagen, stornieren
	repeat [rɪˈpi:t]	Folge-
	extended [ɪkˈstendɪd]	ausgeweitet, erweitert
	surgery [ˈsɜ:dʒəri]	Sprechstunde
	occasional(ly) [əˈkeɪʒənl]	gelegentlich
	pre-booked [ˌpri: ˈbʊkt]	im Voraus gebucht
	duty doctor [ˈdju:ti dɒktə]	diensthabende/r Arzt/Ärztin
	session [ˈseʃn]	Stunde, Sitzung
	extra [ˈekstrə]	zusätzlich

UNIT 3

22	to **find out** [ˌfaɪnd ˈaʊt]	herausfinden
	to **be in a position to do sth** [bi ɪn ə pəˈzɪʃn tə]	in der Lage sein, etw zu tun
	public [ˈpʌblɪk]	öffentlich, staatlich
	insurance coverage [ɪnˈʃʊərəns kʌvərɪdʒ]	Versicherungsschutz
	to **suggest** [səˈdʒest]	nahelegen, andeuten
	to **take care of sb/sth** [teɪk ˈkeər əv]	sich um jdn/etw kümmern
	need [ni:d]	Bedürfnis
	specialist [ˈspeʃəlɪst]	Spezialist/in, Facharzt/ -ärztin; Spezial-, fachärztlich
	to **refer sb to sb** [rɪˈfɜ: tə]	jdn zu jdm überweisen
	straight(away) [streɪt, ˌstreɪtəˈweɪ]	sofort
	whether [ˈweðə]	ob
	bill [bɪl]	Rechnung
	share [ʃeə]	Teil, Anteil
	credit card [ˈkredɪt kɑ:d]	Kreditkarte
	check *AE* [tʃek]	Scheck
	in cash [ɪn ˈkæʃ]	(in) bar
	in full [ɪn ˈfʊl]	vollständig, in voller Höhe
	to **claim sth back** [ˌkleɪm ˈbæk]	etw zurückfordern
	taxpayer [ˈtækspeɪə]	Steuerzahler/in
	charge [tʃɑ:dʒ]	Gebühr(en), Kosten
	free of charge [ˌfri: əf ˈtʃɑ:dʒ]	kostenlos
	medical card [ˈmedɪkl kɑ:d]	Gesundheitskarte
	current [ˈkʌrənt]	aktuell
	prescription charge [prɪˈskrɪpʃn tʃɑ:dʒ]	Rezeptgebühr
	item [ˈaɪtəm]	Artikel
	pharmacy [ˈfɑ:məsi]	Apotheke
	(medical) condition [kənˈdɪʃn]	Leiden, Krankheit
	quite [kwaɪt]	ziemlich
	to **bear** [beə]	tragen
23	**referral** [rɪˈfɜ:rəl]	Überweisung
	in pairs [ɪn ˈpeəz]	paarweise
	state [steɪt]	Staat; staatlich
	walk-in patient [ˈwɔ:k ɪn peɪʃnt]	Patient/in ohne Termin
T	**chest** [tʃest]	Brust
	to **breathe** [bri:ð]	atmen
	stairs *pl* [steəz]	Treppe
	to **be free** [bi ˈfri:]	Zeit haben
	sick [sɪk]	krank
	fever [ˈfi:və]	Fieber
	home visit [ˈhəʊm vɪzɪt]	Hausbesuch
	to **spill sth** [spɪl]	etw verschütten
	boiling [ˈbɔɪlɪŋ]	kochend(heiß)
	happen [ˈhæpən]	passieren, geschehen
	to **hurt** [hɜ:t]	wehtun
	clothes *pl* [kləʊðz]	Kleider
	to **cry** [kraɪ]	weinen, heulen
	sore [sɔ:]	wund, schlimm
	A & E (department) [ˌeɪ ən ˈi:]	Notaufnahme
	to **hurt oneself** [hɜ:t]	sich wehtun, sich verletzen
	painful [ˈpeɪnfl]	schmerzhaft
	to **slip** [slɪp]	ausrutschen
	path [pɑ:θ]	Weg
	swollen [ˈswəʊlən]	geschwollen
	meeting [ˈmi:tɪŋ]	Sitzung, Besprechung, Treffen
	antibiotic [ˌæntibaɪˈɒtɪk]	Antibiotikum
	to **have run out** [həv ˌrʌn ˈaʊt]	aufgebraucht sein
	cough [kɒf]	Husten
	action [ˈækʃn]	Handlung, Maßnahme, Aktion
	to **take action** [ˌteɪk ˈækʃn]	Maßnahme(n) ergreifen
24	**wedding ring** [ˈwedɪŋ rɪŋ]	Ehering
	temperature [ˈtemprətʃə]	Temperatur, Fieber
	to **have a temperature** [həv ə ˈtemprətʃə]	Fieber haben, erhöhte Temperatur haben
	stomach [ˈstʌmək]	Magen, Bauch
	proper(ly) [ˈprɒpə]	richtig, anständig
	although [ɔ:lˈðəʊ]	obwohl
	infection [ɪnˈfekʃn]	Infektion
	medicine [ˈmedsn]	Arzneimittel
	to **get up** [ˌget ˈʌp]	aufstehen
25 T	**treatment room** [ˈtri:tmənt ru:m]	Behandlungsraum

	corridor [ˈkɒrɪdɔː]	Flur
	ID card [ˌaɪ ˈdiː kɑːd]	Personalausweis
	delivery note [dɪˈlɪvəri nəʊt]	Lieferschein
	to **sign** [saɪn]	unterschreiben
	pharmaceutical [ˌfɑːməˈsuːtɪkl]	pharmazeutisch, Pharma-
	storeroom [ˈstɔːruːm]	Lagerraum
	sterilization [sterɪlaɪˈzeɪʃn]	Sterilisation
	floor plan [ˈflɔː plæn]	Grundriss
	to **label** [ˈleɪbl]	etikettieren, bezeichnen
	to **ask for directions** [ˌɑːsk fə dəˈrekʃnz]	nach dem Weg fragen
26	**office equipment** [ˈɒfɪs ɪkwɪpmənt]	Büroausstattung, Bürobedarf
	to **manage** [ˈmænɪdʒ]	verwalten, organisieren
	electronic appointment book [ɪlekˌtrɒnɪk əˈpɔɪntmənt bʊk]	elektronischer Terminkalender
	appointment card [əˈpɔɪntmənt kɑːd]	Terminkarte
	calendar [ˈkælɪndə]	Kalender
	card reader port [ˈkɑːd riːdə pɔːt]	Kartenleseranschluss
	calculator [ˈkælkjuleɪtə]	Taschenrechner
	keyboard [ˈkiːbɔːd]	Tastatur
	label [ˈleɪbl]	Etikett
	printer [ˈprɪntə]	Drucker
	scissors *pl* [ˈsɪzəz]	Schere
	stapler [ˈsteɪplə]	Hefter, Tacker
	cartridge [ˈkɑːtrɪdʒ]	Kartusche, Patrone
	copier [ˈkɒpiə]	Kopierer, Kopiergerät
	to **print** [prɪnt]	drucken, ausdrucken
	document [ˈdɒkjumənt]	Dokument
	to **attach** [əˈtætʃ]	zusammenfügen
	sum [sʌm]	Summe
	to **do sums** [du sʌmz]	rechnen
	copy [ˈkɒpi]	Kopie
	printout [ˈprɪntaʊt]	Ausdruck
27	**order** [ˈɔːdə]	Bestellung, Auftrag
	customer reference number [ˌkʌstəmə ˈrefərəns nʌmbə]	Kundennummer
	pack [pæk]	Packung
	coloured [ˈkʌləd]	bunt, farbig
	staple [ˈsteɪpl]	Heftklammer
	to **come** [kʌm]	*(Waren:)* (es) geben, geliefert werden
	ballpoint pen [ˌbɔːlpɔɪnt ˈpen]	Kugelschreiber
	size [saɪz]	Größe
	in fact [ɪn ˈfækt]	in der Tat, tatsächlich, eigentlich
	special offer [ˌspeʃl ˈɒfə]	Sonderangebot
	actually [ˈæktʃuəli]	wirklich, eigentlich, tatsächlich
	to **work sth out** [ˌwɜːk ˈaʊt]	etw ausrechnen
	total price [ˌtəʊtl ˈpraɪs]	Gesamtpreis
	price [praɪs]	Preis
29	**personal** [ˈpɜːsənl]	persönlich, privat
T	**allergic (to sth)** [əˈlɜːdʒɪk]	allergisch (gegen etw)
	reaction [riˈækʃn]	Reaktion
	kind [kaɪnd]	Art
	drug [drʌg]	Arzneimittel
	anaesthetic [ˌænəsˈθetɪk]	Betäubungsmittel
	medication [ˌmedɪˈkeɪʃn]	Medikamente
	if so [ˈɪf səʊ]	falls ja
	pregnant [ˈpregnənt]	schwanger
	finally [ˈfaɪnəli]	zuletzt, als letztes, schließlich
	nervous [ˈnɜːvəs]	aufgeregt, nervös

UNIT 4

30	**symptom** [ˈsɪmptəm]	Symptom
	gynaecologist [ˌgaɪnəˈkɒlədʒɪst]	Gynäkologe/-in
	paediatrician [ˌpiːdiəˈtrɪʃn]	Kinderarzt/-ärztin
	physiotherapist [ˌfɪziəʊˈθerəpɪst]	Physiotherapeut/-in
	radiologist [ˌreɪdiˈɒlədʒɪst]	Radiologe/-in
	to **break sth** [breɪk]	sich etw brechen
	crutches *pl* [ˈkrʌtʃɪz]	Krücken
	migraine [ˈmiːgreɪn]	Kopfschmerzen, Migräne
	scan [skæn]	(bildgebende) Untersuchung, Computertomographie, Scan
	asthma [ˈæsmə]	Asthma
	to **repair** [rɪˈpeə]	reparieren
	bike [baɪk]	Fahrrad
	cut [kʌt]	Schnitt, Schnittwunde, Schnittverletzung
	close by [kləʊs ˈbaɪ]	nahe gelegen
	deaf [def]	taub
	(ear) wax [wæks]	Ohrenschmalz
	to **syringe** [sɪˈrɪndʒ]	*(Ohren)* ausspülen
	smear test [ˈsmɪə test]	Abstrich
	check-up [ˈtʃekʌp]	(Routine-)Untersuchung
31	to **move** [muːv]	umziehen
	mile [maɪl]	Meile
	tray [treɪ]	Schale
	at all [ət ˈɔːl]	überhaupt
	to **leave school** [liːv ˈskuːl]	von der Schule abgehen
	to **apply for sth** [əˈplaɪ fə]	sich um etw bewerben
32	**throat** [θrəʊt]	Rachen, Hals
	electrocardiograph (ECG) [ɪˌlektrəʊˈkɑːdiəgrɑːf]	Elektrokardiogramm (EKG)
	to **measure** [ˈmeʒə]	messen
	electrical [ɪˈlektrɪkl]	elektrisch
	charge [tʃɑːdʒ]	Ladung
	heart [hɑːt]	Herz

	electroencephalograph (EEG) [ɪˌlektrəʊɪnˈsefələgrɑːf]	Elektroenzephalogramm (EEG)
	activity [ækˈtɪvəti]	Tätigkeit, Aktivität
	brain [breɪn]	Gehirn, Hirn
	trainee [treɪˈniː]	Auszubildende/r
	diagram [ˈdaɪəgræm]	Grafik
	gullet [ˈgʌlɪt]	Speiseröhre
	oesophagus [ɪˈsɒfəgəs]	Oesophagus
	olfactory nerve [ɒlˌfæktri ˈnɜːv]	Geruchsnerv
	windpipe [ˈwɪndpaɪp]	Luftröhre
	trachea [trəˈkiːə]	Trachea
	palate [ˈpælət]	Gaumen
	tongue [tʌŋ]	Zunge
	nasal passage [ˌneɪzl ˈpæsɪdʒ]	Nasengang
T	**air** [eə]	Luft
	to **take in** [ˌteɪk ˈɪn]	*(Luft)* einatmen
	to **pass over sth** [ˌpɑːs ˈəʊvə]	*hier*: über etw streichen
	smell [smel]	Geruch
	back [bæk]	Rückseite, hinterer Teil
	to **carry** [ˈkæri]	befördern, transportieren
	lungs *pl* [lʌŋz]	Lunge
	tooth, teeth [tuːθ, tiːθ]	Zahn, Zähne
	lip [lɪp]	Lippe
	front [frʌnt]	Vorderseite, vorderer Teil
	roof [ruːf]	Dach
	major [ˈmeɪdʒə]	Haupt-
	organ [ˈɔːgən]	Organ
	taste [teɪst]	Geschmack
	to **remember** [rɪˈmembə]	daran denken, nicht vergessen
	to **taste** [teɪst]	schmecken
	anyway [ˈeniweɪ]	also, wie dem auch sei
	to **swallow** [ˈswɒləʊ]	schlucken
	tube [tjuːb]	Röhre
	function [ˈfʌŋkʃn]	Funktion
33	to **make a diagnosis** [ˌmeɪk ə daɪəgˈnəʊsɪs]	eine Diagnose stellen
	sore throat [ˌsɔː ˈθrəʊt]	Halsschmerzen, Halsentzündung
	wide [waɪd]	weit
	trouble [ˈtrʌbl]	Schwierigkeit(en), Problem(e)
	thermometer [θəˈmɒmɪtə]	Thermometer
	to **take one's temperature** [ˌteɪk wʌnz ˈtemprətʃə]	bei jdm Fieber messen
	There we go. [ˌðeə wiː ˈgəʊ]	Los geht's.
	high [haɪ]	*hier:* erhöht
	gland [glænd]	Drüse
	tired [ˈtaɪəd]	müde
	tonsils *pl* [ˈtɒnslz]	Mandeln
	inflamed [ɪnˈfleɪmd]	entzündet
	probably [ˈprɒbəbli]	wahrscheinlich
	tonsillitis [ˌtɒnsəˈlaɪtɪs]	Mandelentzündung
	swab [swɒb]	Abstrich
	to **cause** [kɔːz]	verursachen
	pretty [ˈprɪti]	ziemlich, recht
	to **prescribe** [prɪˈskraɪb]	verschreiben, verordnen
	as far as [əz ˈfɑːr əz]	soweit
	tablet [ˈtæblɪt]	Tablette
	meal [miːl]	Mahlzeit
	plenty of [ˈplenti əv]	viel(e)
	fluids *pl* [ˈfluːɪdz]	Flüssigkeit
	rest [rest]	Ruhe
	to **get some rest** [ˌget səm ˈrest]	sich ausruhen
	sick note [ˈsɪk nəʊt]	Krankschreibung, Attest
	to **seem** [siːm]	scheinen
	neck [nek]	Hals, Nacken
	to **ache** [eɪk]	schmerzen
34	**terrible** [ˈterəbl]	fürchterlich
T	to **sneeze** [sniːz]	niesen
	to **keep doing sth** [ˌkiːp ˈduːɪŋ]	etw die ganze Zeit tun
	blocked [blɒkt]	verstopft
	to **cough** [kɒf]	husten
	to **sit down** [ˌsɪt ˈdaʊn]	sich (hin)setzen
	shoulder [ˈʃəʊldə]	Schulter
	to **take off** [ˌteɪk ˈɒf]	*(Kleidung)* ausziehen
	shirt [ʃɜːt]	Hemd
	to **vomit** [ˈvɒmɪt]	sich erbrechen
	diarrhoea [ˌdaɪəˈrɪə]	Durchfall
	as well [əz ˈwel]	auch, und
	to **notice** [ˈnəʊtɪs]	bemerken
	shy [ʃaɪ]	schüchtern
	Never mind. [ˌnevə ˈmaɪnd]	Macht nichts.
	headache [ˈhedeɪk]	Kopfschmerzen
	rash [ræʃ]	Ausschlag
	spot [spɒt]	Punkt, Fleck
	cold [kəʊld]	Erkältung
	poisoning [ˈpɔɪzənɪŋ]	Vergiftung
	food poisoning [ˈfuːd pɔɪzənɪŋ]	Lebensmittelvergiftung
	flu [fluː]	Grippe
	measles *pl* [ˈmiːzlz]	Masern
	to **agree** [əˈgriː]	zustimmen
	to **disagree** [ˌdɪsəˈgriː]	nicht zustimmen
35	to **examine** [ɪgˈzæmɪn]	untersuchen
T	to **roll up** [ˌrəʊl ˈʌp]	*(Ärmel)* hochkrempeln
	sleeve [sliːv]	Ärmel
	chain [tʃeɪn]	Kette
	screwdriver [ˈskruːdraɪvə]	Schraubenzieher
	to **slip** [slɪp]	abrutschen
	bandage [ˈbændɪdʒ]	Verband
	to **heal** [hiːl]	heilen, verheilen
	stitch [stɪtʃ]	Stich
	recently [ˈriːsntli]	in letzter Zeit

	to remember (sth) [rɪˈmembə]	sich (an etw) erinnern
	to disinfect [ˌdɪsɪnˈfekt]	desinfizieren
	to hold out [ˌhəʊld ˈaʊt]	hinhalten
	to take (it in) turns in doing sth [ˌteɪk ˈtɜːnz ɪn]	etw abwechselnd tun
	to consult [kənˈsʌlt]	konsultieren; beraten
	examination/exam [ɪɡˌzæmɪˈneɪʃn, ɪɡˈzæm]	Untersuchung
	dressing [ˈdresɪŋ]	Verband
	backache [ˈbækeɪk]	Rückenschmerzen
	stomach ache [ˈstʌməkeɪk]	Bauchschmerzen
	earache [ˈɪəreɪk]	Ohrenschmerzen
	to keep food down [ˌkiːp ˈfuːd daʊn]	Essen bei sich behalten
	joint [dʒɔɪnt]	Gelenk
37	**article** [ˈɑːtɪkl]	Artikel
	disease [dɪˈziːz]	Erkrankung, Krankheit
	heart disease [ˈhɑːt dɪziːz]	Herzerkrankung
	heart attack [ˈhɑːt ətæk]	Herzinfarkt
	to die (from sth) [daɪ]	(an etw) sterben
	to recognise [ˈrekəgnaɪz]	erkennen
	middle-aged [ˌmɪdlˈeɪdʒd]	mittleren Alters
	overweight [ˌəʊvəˈweɪt]	übergewichtig
	per cent [pə ˈsent]	Prozent
	compared with [kəmˈpeəd wɪð]	verglichen mit
	mild [maɪld]	leicht
	dizzy [ˈdɪzi]	schwindlig
	pulse [pʌls]	Puls
	to take sb's pulse [ˌteɪk ˈpʌls]	jds Puls messen
	heart rate [ˈhɑːt reɪt]	Puls, Herzfrequenz
	to carry out [ˌkæri ˈaʊt]	durchführen
	ambulance [ˈæmbjələns]	Rettungswagen
	to call [kɔːl]	rufen
	view [vjuː]	Ansicht
	consultant [kənˈsʌltənt]	Facharzt/-ärztin
	cardiologist [ˌkɑːdɪˈɒlədʒɪst]	Kardiologe/-in
	director [dəˈrektə]	Direktor/in
	foundation [faʊnˈdeɪʃn]	Stiftung
	mainly [ˈmeɪnli]	hauptsächlich
	coronary heart disease [ˌkɒrənrɪ ˈhɑːt dɪziːz]	koronare Herzerkrankung
	to believe [bɪˈliːv]	glauben
	stressed [strest]	gestresst
	overworked [ˌəʊvəˈwɜːkt]	überarbeitet
	to deal with sth [ˈdiːl wɪð]	mit etw zu tun haben
	risk [rɪsk]	Risiko, Gefahr
	factor [ˈfæktə]	Faktor
	obesity [əʊˈbiːsəti]	Fettleibigkeit
	to affect [əˈfekt]	betreffen
	additional [əˈdɪʃənl]	zusätzlich, Zusatz-
	development [dɪˈveləpmənt]	Entwicklung
	diabetes [ˌdaɪəˈbiːtiːz]	Diabetes
	to be at risk [bi ət ˈrɪsk]	gefährdet sein
	depression [dɪˈpreʃn]	Depression
	menopause [ˈmenəpɔːz]	Wechseljahre, Menopause
	oestrogen [ˈiːstrədʒən]	Östrogen
	to present [prɪˈzent]	darstellen
	significant [sɪɡˈnɪfɪkənt]	bedeutend, erheblich
	to develop [dɪˈveləp]	entwickeln
	cardiovascular [ˌkɑːdiəʊˈvæskjələ]	Herz-Kreislauf-, kardiovaskulär
	candidate [ˈkændɪdət]	Kandidat/in
	cause [kɔːz]	Ursache
	to design [dɪˈzaɪn]	gestalten, entwerfen
	leaflet [ˈliːflət]	Broschüre, Merkblatt
	warning signal [ˈwɔːnɪŋ sɪɡnəl]	Warnsignal

UNIT 5

38	**examination gloves** *pl* [ɪɡˌzæmɪˈneɪʃn glʌvz]	Untersuchungshandschuhe
	hypodermic (syringe) [ˌhaɪpəˈdɜːmɪk]	Injektionsspritze
	disinfectant [ˌdɪsɪnˈfektənt]	Desinfektionsmittel
	elastic [ɪˈlæstɪk]	elastisch
	bandage [ˈbændɪdʒ]	Binde, Bandage
	tourniquet [ˈtʊənɪkeɪ]	Stauschlauch, Venenstauer
	tweezers *pl* [ˈtwiːzəz]	Pinzette
	gauze [gɔːz]	Gaze, Verbandmull
	cotton [ˈkɒtn]	Baumwolle
	swab [swɒb]	Tupfer
	scalpel [ˈskælpəl]	Skalpell
	stethoscope [ˈsteθəskəʊp]	Stethoskop
	otoscope [ˈəʊtəskəʊp]	Ohrenspiegel, Otoskop
	blood-pressure cuff [ˈblʌd preʃə kʌf]	Blutdruckmanschette
	needle [ˈniːdl]	Nadel
	needle-holder [ˈniːdl həʊldə]	Nadelhalter
	needle-thread combination [ˌniːld ˈθred kɒmbɪneɪʃn]	Nadel-Faden-Kombination
39	**piece of equipment** [ˌpiːs əv ɪˈkwɪpmənt]	Gerät, Utensil
	wound [wuːnd]	Wunde
	to dress [dres]	*(Wunde)* verbinden
	to stitch [stɪtʃ]	nähen
	to extract [ɪkˈstrækt]	herausziehen
	to inject [ɪnˈdʒekt]	injizieren
	to protect [prəˈtekt]	schützen
	heartbeat [ˈhɑːtbiːt]	Herzschlag
	sprain [spreɪn]	Verstauchung
	splinter [ˈsplɪntə]	Splitter
	skin [skɪn]	Haut
	broken glass [ˌbrəʊkən ˈglɑːs]	Glasscherbe(n)
	to give a local anaesthetic [gɪv ə ˌləʊkl ænəsˈθetɪk]	örtlich betäuben

	to **take stitches out** [ˌteɪk ˈstɪtʃɪz aʊt]	Fäden ziehen
	to **tie off stitches** [taɪ ˌɒf ˈstɪtʃɪz]	Fäden vernähen
T	**sting** [stɪŋ]	schmerzen, brennen
	to **take effect** [teɪk ɪˈfekt]	wirken
	to **get sth ready** [get ˈredi]	etw vorbereiten
41	**immunization** [ˌɪmjunaɪˈzeɪʃn]	Schutzimpfung, Immunisierung
	jacket [ˈdʒækɪt]	Jacke
	tight [taɪt]	eng, fest
	plaster [ˈplɑːstə]	Pflaster
	actual [ˈæktʃuəl]	wirklich, tatsächlich
	to **compare** [kəmˈpeə]	vergleichen
T	**hepatitis** [ˌhepəˈtaɪtɪs]	Hepatitis
	sight [saɪt]	Anblick
	glad [glæd]	froh
	cottonwool [ˌkɒtnˈwʊl]	Watte
42	**reading** [ˈriːdɪŋ]	Wert, Messwert
	to **beat** [biːt]	schlagen
	to **rise** [raɪz]	steigen, ansteigen
	to **record** [rɪˈkɔːd]	aufzeichnen, festhalten
	mercury [ˈmɜːkjəri]	Quecksilber
	artery [ˈɑːtəri]	Arterie
	muscle [ˈmʌsl]	Muskel
	to **contract** [kənˈtrækt]	sich zusammenziehen
	systolic [sɪˈstɒlɪk]	systolisch
	to **rest** [rest]	ruhen
	diastolic [daɪəˈstɒlɪk]	diastolisch
	steadily [ˈstedɪli]	kontinuierlich, stetig
	increasing [ɪnˈkriːsɪŋ]	zunehmend
	stiffness [ˈstɪfnəs]	Steifheit
	long-term [ˌlɒŋˈtɜːm]	langfristig
	build-up [ˈbɪldʌp]	Aufbau
	plaque [plɑːk]	Ablagerung(en)
	frequent [ˈfriːkwənt]	häufig
	cardiac [ˈkɑːdɪak]	Herz-
	vascular [ˈvæskjʊlə]	Gefäß-
	to **change** [tʃeɪndʒ]	(sich) verändern, (sich) ändern
	change [tʃeɪndʒ]	Änderung, Veränderung
	exercise [ˈeksəsaɪz]	Bewegung, (Ausgleichs-) Sport
	aged [eɪdʒd]	im Alter von
	to **monitor** [ˈmɒnɪtə]	überwachen
	high blood pressure [haɪ ˈblʌd preʃə]	Bluthochdruck
	not necessarily [nɒt ˌnesəˈserəli]	nicht unbedingt
	likely [ˈlaɪkli]	wahrscheinlich
	almost [ˈɔːlməʊst]	fast, beinah
	lifestyle [ˈlaɪfstaɪl]	Lebensweise
	repeated [rɪˈpiːtɪd]	wiederholt
	to **seek** [siːk]	suchen
	immediate(ly) [ɪˈmiːdiət]	unverzüglich, sofortig
	hypertensive crisis [haɪpəˌtensɪv ˈkraɪsɪs]	hypertensive Krise
	category [ˈkætəgəri]	Klasse, Kategorie
	upper [ˈʌpə]	obere/r/s
	value [ˈvæljuː]	Wert
	lower [ˈləʊə]	untere/r/s
	prehypertension [ˌpriːˌhaɪpəˈtenʃən]	Prähypertonie
	hypertension [ˌhaɪpəˈtenʃn]	Hypertonie
	stage [steɪdʒ]	Stufe
	to **make a difference** [ˌmeɪk ə ˈdɪfrəns]	etwas/viel ausmachen
	extreme(ly) [ɪkˈstriːm]	extrem
43	**bulb** [bʌlb]	Ballon
	cuff [kʌf]	Manschette
	gauge [geɪdʒ]	Messgerät, *hier:* Manometer
	valve [vælv]	Ventil
	order [ˈɔːdə]	Reihenfolge
	to **continue to do sth** [kənˈtɪnjuː tə]	etw weiter(hin) tun
	to **deflate sth** [dɪˈfleɪt]	Luft aus etw lassen
	sound [saʊnd]	Geräusch
	to **fade** [feɪd]	schwächer werden, verklingen
	to **double-check** [ˌdʌblˈtʃek]	nochmals kontrollieren
	accuracy [ˈækjərəsi]	Genauigkeit
	to **place** [pleɪs]	platzieren
	to **locate** [ləʊˈkeɪt]	ausfindig machen
	brachial artery [ˌbreɪkiəl ˈɑːtəri]	Oberarmarterie
	to **fit** [fɪt]	passen, sitzen
	snugly [ˈsnʌgli]	eng, wie angegossen
	to **inflate** [ɪnˈfleɪt]	aufpumpen
	to **pump** [pʌmp]	pumpen
	until [ənˈtɪl]	bis
	blood flow [ˈblʌd fləʊ]	Blutstom, Durchblutung
	to **allow sth for sth** [əˈlaʊ fə]	etw für etw vorsehen
	clothing [ˈkləʊðɪŋ]	Kleidung, Bekleidung
	to **get in the way of sth** [ˌget ɪn ðə ˈweɪ əv]	einer Sache im Wege sein
	to **position** [pəˈzɪʃn]	positionieren
45	**video conferencing** [ˈvɪdiəʊ kɒnfərənsɪŋ]	Videokonferenz(schaltung)
	remote [rɪˈməʊt]	fern, Fern-
	medical consultation [ˌmedɪkl kɒnslˈteɪʃn]	medizinische Beratung
	to **connect** [kəˈnekt]	verbinden
	to **take off** [ˌteɪk ˈɒf]	durchstarten, sich verbreiten
	Scotland [ˈskɒtlənd]	Schottland
	royal [ˈrɔɪəl]	königlich
	infirmary [ɪnˈfɜːmri]	Krankenhaus
	to **conduct** [kənˈdʌkt]	durchführen
	experiment [ɪkˈsperɪmənt]	Versuch, Experiment
	telemedicine [ˈteləmedsən]	Telemedizin

trial [ˈtraɪəl] — Test, Versuch
face-to-face [ˌfeɪs tə ˈfeɪs] — direkt, persönlich
technology [tekˈnɒlədʒi] — Technik, Technologie
to **present** [prɪˈzent] — zeigen, präsentieren
life-size [!laɪfsaɪz] — lebensgroß
image [ˈɪmɪdʒ] — Bild
high-definition [ˌhaɪ ˌdefɪˈnɪʃn] — hochauflösend
as if [əz ˈɪf] — als ob
across sth [əˈkrɒs] — auf der anderen Seite von etw

booth [ˌdʒæki ˈbuːð] — Kabine
device [dɪˈvaɪs] — Gerät
whole [həʊl] — ganz
setup [ˈsetʌp] — Aufbau, Anordnung, Einrichtung

broadband [ˈbrɔːdbænd] — Breitband
network [ˈnetwɜːk] — Netzwerk
experience [ɪkˈspɪəriəns] — Erlebnis
close to life [ˌkləʊs tə ˈlaɪf] — lebensnah
to **volunteer** [ˌvɒlənˈtɪə] — sich (freiwillig) zur Verfügung stellen

stage [steɪdʒ] — Phase, Abschnitt
to **move** [muːv] — verlegen
site [saɪt] — Standort
community [kəˈmjuːnəti] — Gemeinde
hands-on [ˌhændz ˈɒn] — praktisch, direkt
police station [pəˈliːs steɪʃn] — Polizeiwache
to **succeed** [səkˈsiːd] — Erfolg haben, erfolgreich sein

to **create** [kriˈeɪt] — schaffen
to **set up** [ˌset ˈʌp] — einrichten, aufbauen
sponsored [ˈspɒnsəd] — gefördert
pilot trial [ˈpaɪlət traɪəl] — Pilotversuch, Pilotprojekt
to **run sth** [rʌn] — etw leiten, etw führen
ongoing [ˈɒngəʊɪŋ] — laufend, andauernd
across … [əˈkrɒs] — im gesamten …
lesson [ˈlesn] — Lehre, Lektion
jigsaw puzzle [ˈdʒɪgsɔː pʌzl] — Puzzle
special [ˈspeʃl] — speziell, besondere/r/s
summary [ˈsʌməri] — Zusammenfassung
recommendation [ˌrekəmenˈdeɪʃn] — Empfehlung
advantage [ədˈvɑːntɪdʒ] — Vorteil, Vorzug
disadvantage [ˌdɪsədˈvɑːntɪdʒ] — Nachteil

UNIT 6

46 T
smallpox [ˈsmɔːlpɒks] — Pocken
vaccination [ˌvæksɪˈneɪʃn] — Impfung, Schutzimpfung
scary [ˈskeəri] — furchteinflößend, unheimlich
kid [kɪd] — Kind
pelvic [ˈpelvɪk] — Becken-
pelvic examination [ˌpelvɪk ɪgzæmɪˈneɪʃn] — gynäkologische Untersuchung
to **renew** [rɪˈnjuː] — erneuern
to **phone in** [ˌfəʊn ˈɪn] — anrufen
urine sample [ˈjʊərɪn sɑːmpl] — Urinprobe
to **take a day off work** [teɪk ə deɪ ˌɒf ˈwɜːk] — sich einen Tag frei nehmen
to **pick up** [ˌpɪk ˈʌp] — abholen
serious [ˈsɪəriəs] — schwer, ernst
beach [biːtʃ] — Strand
tetanus [ˈtetənəs] — Tetanus
awful(ly) [ˈɔːfl] — schrecklich, fürchterlich
to **spread** [spred] — verbreiten
germ [dʒɜːm] — Keim, Bakterie

to **be scared of sth** [bi ˈskeəd əv] — vor etw Angst haben

47
difficulty [ˈdɪfɪkəlti] — Schwierigkeit
cultural [ˈkʌltʃərəl] — kulturell
physical [ˈfɪzɪkl] — körperlich
mental [ˈmentl] — geistig
suggestion [səˈdʒestʃən] — Vorschlag
hearing aid [ˈhɪərɪŋ eɪd] — Hörgerät
wheelchair [ˈwiːltʃeə] — Rollstuhl
pushchair [ˈpʊʃtʃeə] — Buggy *(Kinderwagen)*
Chinese [tʃaɪˈniːz] — chinesisch
toy [tɔɪ] — Spielzeug
to **undress** [ˌʌnˈdres] — sich ausziehen
explanation [ˌekspləˈneɪʃn] — Erklärung, Erläuterung
disabled [dɪsˈeɪbld] — behindert
partially [ˈpɑːʃəli] — teilweise, zum Teil
scale [skeɪl] — Skala
tense [tens] — angespannt
worried [ˈwʌrid] — besorgt, beunruhigt
dental [ˈdentl] — Zahn-
to **take an exam** [ˌteɪk ən ɪgˈzæm] — eine Prüfung machen
job interview [ˈdʒɒb ɪntəvjuː] — Vorstellungsgespräch
to **express** [ɪkˈspres] — ausdrücken
anxiety [æŋˈzaɪəti] — Angst, Ängstlichkeit, Besorgnis

to **be afraid of sb/sth** [bi əˈfreɪd əv] — sich vor jdm/etw fürchten
to **be anxious about sth** [bi ˈæŋkʃəs əbaʊt] — sich um/wegen etw Sorgen machen
to **feel uncomfortable** [ˌfiːl ʌnˈkʌmftəbl] — sich unwohl fühlen
to **worry about sth** [ˈwʌri əbaʊt] — sich um etw Sorgen machen
paragraph [ˈpærəgrɑːf] — *(Text:)* Absatz
heading [ˈhedɪŋ] — Überschrift
fear (of sth) [fɪə] — Furcht, Angst (vor etw)
news *pl* [njuːz] — Neuigkeiten, Nachrichten
death [deθ] — Tod
poor [pʊə] — schlecht, dürftig

	infection [ɪnˈfekʃn]	Ansteckung
48	to **hate** [heɪt]	hassen, überhaupt nicht mögen
	atmosphere [ˈætməsfɪə]	Atmosphäre, Stimmung
	to **smell (of sth)** [smel]	(nach etw) riechen
	to **suffer from sth** [ˈsʌfə frəm]	an etw leiden
	cancer [ˈkænsə]	Krebs *(Krankheit)*
	seriously [ˈsɪəriəsli]	schwer, ernsthaft
	coldness [ˈkəʊldnəs]	Kälte
	trained [treɪnd]	geschult, ausgebildet
	objective [əbˈdʒektɪv]	objektiv
	distant [ˈdɪstənt]	distanziert
	sheet of paper [ˌʃiːt əf ˈpeɪpə]	Blatt Papier
	to **associate sb with sth** [əˈsəʊʃieɪt wɪð]	jdn mit etw in Verbindung bringen
	to **involve** [ɪnˈvɒlv]	mit sich bringen, einschließen
	helpless [ˈhelpləs]	hilflos
	rather [ˈrɑːðə]	eher, lieber
	truth [truːθ]	Wahrheit
	to **catch sth** [kætʃ]	sich mit etw anstecken
	unfriendly [ʌnˈfrendli]	unfreundlich
	to **feel comfortable** [ˌfiːl ˈkʌmftəbl]	sich wohlfühlen
49	**relaxing** [rɪˈlæksɪŋ]	entspannend
	fully [ˈfʊli]	vollständig
	foot spa [ˈfʊt spɑː]	Fußbad
	to **massage** [ˈmæsɑːʒ]	massieren
	aromatherapy [əˌrəʊməˈθerəpi]	Aromatherapie
	candle [ˈkændl]	Kerze
	children's corner [ˌtʃɪldrənz ˈkɔːnə]	Spielecke
	nowadays [ˈnaʊədeɪz]	heutzutage
	improvement [ɪmˈpruːvmənt]	Verbesserung
	invasive [ɪnˈveɪsɪv]	invasiv
T	**medicine** [ˈmedsn]	Medizin
	painless [ˈpeɪnləs]	schmerzlos
	to **expect (sb to do sth)** [ɪkˈspekt]	erwarten (dass jd etw tut)
	benefit [ˈbenɪfɪt]	Nutzen, Vorteil
	to **suppose** [səˈpəʊz]	annehmen, glauben
	progress [ˈprəʊgres]	Fortschritt
	to **trust** [trʌst]	vertrauen
	rushed [rʌʃt]	gehetzt
	to **bet** [bet]	wetten
	soft [sɒft]	leise
	to **burn a candle** [ˌbɜːn ə ˈkændl]	eine Kerze verwenden, brennen lassen
	massage [ˈmæsɑːʒ]	Massage
	to **relieve** [rɪˈliːv]	lindern, abbauen
	reassurance [ˌriːəˈʃʊərəns]	Beruhigung
50	to **lie around** [ˌlaɪ əˈraʊnd]	herumliegen
51	**distress** [dɪˈstres]	Kummer, Sorge, Verzweiflung
	to **calm** [kɑːm]	beruhigen
	to **reassure** [ˌriːəˈʃʊə]	beruhigen
T	**completely** [kəmˈpliːtli]	völlig, vollkommen
	breast [brest]	Brust
	to **stand** [stænd]	stehen
	self-exam [ˈself ɪgzæm]	Selbstuntersuchung
	present [ˈpreznt]	anwesend
	to **lie down** [ˌlaɪ ˈdaʊn]	sich hinlegen
	cell [sel]	Zelle
	cervix [ˈsɜːvɪks]	Gebärmutterhals
	tiny [ˈtaɪni]	klein
	wooden stick [ˌwʊdn ˈstɪk]	Holzstab
	brush [brʌʃ]	Bürste, Pinsel
	absolutely [ˈæbsəluːtli]	völlig, absolut, ganz
	internal [ɪnˈtɜːnl]	innere/r/s
	discomfort [dɪsˈkʌmfət]	Unbehagen, leichter Schmerz
	right away [raɪt əˈweɪ]	sofort
	in detail [ɪn ˈdiːteɪl]	im Einzelnen, detailliert
	gentle [ˈdʒentl]	behutsam
	perfectly [ˈpɜːfɪktli]	völlig
	human [ˈhjuːmən]	human, menschlich
	papilloma virus [pæpəˈləʊmə vaɪrəs]	Papillomvirus
	reduction [rɪˈdʌkʃn]	Rückgang
	to **make sth up** [ˌmeɪk ˈʌp]	sich etw ausdenken, etw erfinden
52	**dosage** [ˈdəʊsɪdʒ]	Dosierung
	instruction(s) [ɪnˈstrʌkʃn]	Anleitung
	unless [ənˈles]	wenn nicht
	otherwise [ˈʌðəwaɪz]	anders
	once [wʌns]	einmal
	twice [twaɪs]	zweimal
	pill [pɪl]	Pille
	capsule [ˈkæpsjuːl]	Kapsel
	empty [ˈempti]	leer
	to **dissolve** [dɪˈzɒlv]	auflösen
	to **allow to dissolve** [əˌlaʊ tə dɪˈzɒlv]	zergehen lassen
	side effect [ˈsaɪd ɪfekt]	Nebenwirkung
	minority [maɪˈnɒrəti]	Minderzahl
	drowsiness [ˈdraʊzinəs]	Schläfrigkeit
	nausea [ˈnɔːziə]	Übelkeit
	stomach complaints *pl* [ˈstʌmək kəmpleɪnts]	Magenbeschwerden
	blurred vision [ˌblɜːd ˈvɪʒn]	verschwommenes Sehen
	to **collect** [kəˈlekt]	abholen
	to **outline** [ˈaʊtlaɪn]	(kurz) darstellen, umreißen
55	**presentation** [ˌpreznˈteɪʃn]	Präsentation, Vortrag
	to **train** [treɪn]	eine Ausbildung machen
	social care [ˌsəʊʃl ˈkeə]	Sozialfürsorge, Sozialdienste
	relationship [rɪˈleɪʃnʃɪp]	Beziehung, Verhältnis
	to **avoid** [əˈvɔɪd]	vermeiden
	talk [tɔːk]	Vortrag

	honest ['ɒnɪst]	ehrlich, aufrichtig
	client ['klaɪənt]	Klient/in, Kunde/Kundin
	to **take care of sb** [teɪk 'keər əv]	auf jdn aufpassen, sich um jdn kümmern
	patient ['peɪʃnt]	geduldig
	success [sək'ses]	Erfolg

T	to **rely on sth** [rɪ'laɪ ɒn]	auf etw angewiesen sein
	trust [trʌst]	Vertrauen
	understanding [ˌʌndə'stændɪŋ]	Verständnis
	task [tɑːsk]	Aufgabe
	dignity ['dɪgnəti]	Würde
	therefore ['ðeəfɔː]	daher, deshalb
	warmth [wɔːmθ]	Wärme
	angry ['æŋgri]	ungehalten, wütend
	frustrated [frʌ'streɪtɪd]	frustriert
	essential [ɪ'senʃl]	wesentlich, notwendig
	to **react** [ri'ækt]	reagieren
	to **take sth personally** [ˌteɪk 'pɜːsənəli]	etw persönlich nehmen
	ill-tempered [ˌɪl'tempəd]	griesgrämig, verärgert
	lonely ['ləʊnli]	einsam
	helplessness ['helpləsnəs]	Hilflosigkeit
	weakness ['wiːknəs]	Schwäche
	lazy ['leɪzi]	faul
	simply ['sɪmpli]	(ganz) einfach
	to **reduce** [rɪ'djuːs]	verringern
	self-respect [ˌself rɪ'spekt]	Selbstachtung
	self-esteem [ˌself ɪ'stiːm]	Selbstwertgefühl
	to **rush around** [ˌrʌʃ ə'raʊnd]	umherhetzen
	honesty ['ɒnəsti]	Ehrlichkeit, Aufrichtigkeit
	to **apologize** [ə'pɒlədʒaɪz]	sich entschuldigen
	to **put things right** [pʊt ˌθɪŋz 'raɪt]	Abhilfe schaffen
	to **take time off** [teɪk taɪm 'ɒf]	sich freinehmen, sich Zeit nehmen
	to **enjoy** [ɪn'dʒɔɪ]	genießen, gern tun
	manager ['mænɪdʒə]	Geschäftsführer/in

UNIT 7

56	**nutrition** [nju'trɪʃn]	Ernährung
	healthy ['helθi]	gesund
	diet ['daɪət]	Ernährung, Kost
	scientific [ˌsaɪən'tɪfɪk]	wissenschaftlich
	study ['stʌdi]	Untersuchung, Studie
	obese [əʊ'biːs]	fettleibig
	concentration [ˌkɒnsn'treɪʃn]	Konzentration
	to **be badly behaved** [bi ˌbædli bɪ'heɪvd]	sich schlecht benehmen, unartig sein
	to **contain** [kən'teɪn]	enthalten
	plum [plʌm]	Pflaume
	percentage [pə'sentɪdʒ]	Anteil, Prozentsatz
	calorie ['kæləri]	Kalorie
	intake ['ɪnteɪk]	Zufuhr
	carbohydrates *pl* [ˌkɑːbəʊ'haɪdreɪts]	Kohlenhydrate
57	**chart** [tʃɑːt]	Grafik
	fat [fæt]	Fett
	oil [ɔɪl]	Öl
	meat [miːt]	Fleisch
	cold cut ['kəʊld kʌt]	Aufschnitt
	dairy products ['deəri prɒdʌkts]	Molkereiprodukte, Milchprodukte
	vegetables *pl* ['vedʒtəblz]	Gemüse
	salad ['sæləd]	Salat
	cereal ['sɪəriəl]	Getreide, Getreideflocken
	salt [sɒlt]	Salz
	cream [kriːm]	Sahne
	sugar ['ʃʊgə]	Zucker
	biscuit ['bɪskɪt]	Keks
	bread roll ['bred rəʊl]	Brötchen
	juice [dʒuːs]	Saft
	salmon ['sæmən]	Lachs
	chicken ['tʃɪkɪn]	Huhn
	sausage ['sɒsɪdʒ]	(Brat-)Wurst
	onion ['ʌnjən]	Zwiebel
	maple syrup [ˌmeɪpl 'sɪrəp]	Ahornsirup
	to **consume** [kən'sjuːm]	verzehren
	amount [ə'maʊnt]	Menge

T	**pregnancy** ['pregnənsi]	Schwangerschaft
	to **recommend** [ˌrekə'mend]	empfehlen
	folic acid [ˌfəʊlɪk 'æsɪd]	Folsäure
	cabbage ['kæbɪdʒ]	Kohl
	spinach ['spɪnɪtʃ]	Spinat
	fibre ['faɪbə]	Ballaststoff
	high-fibre ['haɪfaɪbə]	ballaststoffreich
	vitamin ['vɪtəmɪn]	Vitamin
	to **harm** [hɑːm]	schädigen, schaden
	foetus ['fiːtəs]	Fötus
	smoker ['sməʊkə]	Raucher/in
	vegetable oil ['vedʒtəbl ɔɪl]	Pflanzenöl
	olive ['ɒlɪv]	Olive
	rapeseed *BE*, **canola** *AE* ['reɪpsiːd, kə'nəʊlə]	Raps
	animal ['ænɪml]	tierisch
	yoghurt ['jɒgət]	Joghurt
	beef [biːf]	Rind(fleisch)
	pork [pɔːk]	Schwein(efleisch)
	to **increase** [ɪn'kriːs]	erhöhen
	cholesterol [kə'lestərɒl]	Cholesterin
	cholesterol level [kə'lestərɒl levl]	Cholesterinspiegel
	harmful ['hɑːmfl]	schädlich
	to **be high in sth** [bi 'haɪ ɪn]	einen hohen Anteil von etw haben
	coconut ['kəʊkənʌt]	Kokosnuss
	coconut oil ['kəʊkənʌt ɔɪl]	Kokosöl
	palm oil ['pɑːm ɔɪl]	Palmöl
	saturated fats *pl* [ˌsætʃəreɪtɪd 'fæts]	gesättigte Fettsäuren

	to **limit** ['lɪmɪt]	begrenzen, beschränken
	baby food ['beɪbi fu:d]	Babynahrung
	unsweetened [ˌʌn'swi:tnd]	ungesüßt
58	**grain** [greɪn]	Korn, Getreide
	substance ['sʌbstəns]	Stoff, Substanz
	skimmed milk [ˌskɪmd 'mɪlk]	entrahmte Milch
	full fat milk [fʊl ˌfæt 'mɪlk]	Vollmilch
	killer ['kɪlə]	Todesursache
	jar [dʒɑ:]	Glas
	to **prepare** [prɪ'peə]	*(Essen)* kochen, zubereiten
	fresh [freʃ]	frisch
	honey ['hʌni]	Honig
	condition [kən'dɪʃn]	Zustand
	to **improve** [ɪm'pru:v]	(sich) bessern, verbessern
59	to **diagnose sb with sth** ['daɪəgnəʊz wɪð]	etw *(Krankheit)* bei jdm feststellen
	commonly ['kɒmənli]	häufig, gewöhnlich
	contagious [kən'teɪdʒəs]	ansteckend
	genetic [dʒə'netɪk]	genetisch, erblich
	environmental [ɪnˌvaɪrən'mentl]	Umwelt-
	type [taɪp]	Typ
	equally ['i:kwəli]	gleich, gleichermaßen
	to **lead** [li:d]	führen
	insulin ['ɪnsjʊlɪn]	Insulin
	coach [kəʊtʃ]	Reisebus
	gold medal [ˌgəʊld 'medl]	Goldmedaille
	rower ['rəʊə]	Ruderer/-in
	to **do exercise** [du: 'eksəsaɪz]	sich bewegen, Sport treiben
	to **advise** [əd'vaɪz]	raten, beraten
	flu jab ['flu: dʒæb]	Grippe(schutz)impfung
	blood glucose control ['blʌd glu:kəʊs kəntrəʊl]	Blutzuckerregulation
	to **put sb at risk** [ˌpʊt ət 'rɪsk]	jdn einem Risiko aussetzen
	blood glucose level ['blʌd glu:kəʊs levl]	Blutzuckerspiegel
	sugary ['ʃʊgəri]	süß, zuckerhaltig
	confectionery foods *pl* [kən'fekʃənəri fu:dz]	Süßwaren
	weight [weɪt]	Gewicht
	to **lose weight** [ˌlu:z 'weɪt]	abnehmen
60	**opposite** ['ɒpəzɪt]	Gegenteil
	incorrect [ˌɪnkə'rekt]	falsch
	underweight [ˌʌndə'weɪt]	untergewichtig
	to **decrease** [dɪ'kri:s]	abnehmen, sinken
	unhealthy [ʌn'helθi]	ungesund
	to **estimate** ['estɪmeɪt]	schätzen
	worldwide ['wɜ:ldwaɪd]	weltweit
	to **be equal to sth** [bi 'i:kwəl tə]	entsprechen
	population [ˌpɒpju'leɪʃn]	Bevölkerung
	to **account for sth** [ə'kaʊnt fə]	etw ausmachen
	to **result in sth** [rɪ'zʌlt ɪn]	etw zur Folge haben
	death [deθ]	Todesfall
	global ['gləʊbl]	weltweit, global
	economic [ˌi:kə'nɒmɪk]	wirtschaftlich, ökonomisch
	infectious [ɪn'fekʃəs]	ansteckend
	diabetic [ˌdaɪə'betɪk]	Diabetes-
	covered in sth ['kʌvəd ɪn]	*hier:* mit etw überzogen
61	**Polish** ['pəʊlɪʃ]	polnisch
	national ['næʃnəl]	Staatsbürger/in
	to **pay attention to sth** [ˌpeɪ ə'tenʃn tə]	auf etw achten
	self-care [ˌself 'keə]	Eigenfürsorge
	crazy ['kreɪzi]	verrückt
	chest infection ['tʃest ɪnfekʃn]	Lungeninfekt
	progressive [prə'gresɪv]	fortschreitend
	damage ['dæmɪdʒ]	Schaden, Schäden
	nerve [nɜ:v]	Nerv
	support [sə'pɔ:t]	Hilfe, Unterstützung
63	**chef** [ʃef]	Koch/Köchin, Küchenchef/in
	high-profile [ˌhaɪ 'prəʊfaɪl]	öffentlichkeitswirksam
	campaign [kæm'peɪn]	Kampagne
	to **introduce** [ˌɪntrə'dju:s]	einführen
	eating habits *pl* ['i:tɪŋ hæbɪts]	Essgewohnheiten
	to **serve** [sɜ:v]	servieren
	programme ['prəʊgræm]	(Fernseh-, Radio-)Sendung
	school dinner [ˌsku:l 'dɪnə]	Schulessen
	chips *BE* [tʃɪps]	Pommes frites
	to **ban** [bæn]	verbieten
	crisps *BE* [krɪsps]	Chips
	carbonated ['kɑ:bəneɪtɪd]	mit Kohlensäure
	award-winning [ə'wɔ:d wɪnɪŋ]	preisgekrönt
	TV show [ˌti: 'vi: ʃəʊ]	Fernsehsendung, -serie
	viewer ['vju:ə]	Zuschauer/in
	to **report** [rɪ'pɔ:t]	berichten
	government ['gʌvənmənt]	Regierung
	financial injection [faɪˌnænʃl ɪn'dʒekʃn]	finanzielle Unterstützung, Finanzspritze
	introduction [ˌɪntrə'dʌkʃn]	Einführung
	guidelines *pl* ['gaɪdlaɪnz]	Richtlinien
	despite [dɪ'spaɪt]	trotz
	victory ['vɪktəri]	Sieg
	popularity [ˌpɒpju'lærəti]	Beliebtheit
	drop [drɒp]	Rückgang
	growing ['grəʊɪŋ]	wachsend, zunehmend, steigend
	black market [ˌblæk 'mɑ:kɪt]	Schwarzmarkt
	non-nutritional [ˌnɒn nju'trɪʃənl]	nährwertlos
	burger van ['bɜ:gə væn]	Imbisswagen
	to **pass sth** [pɑ:s]	etw reichen
	gate [geɪt]	Tor

	fizzy drink ['fɪzi drɪŋk]	kohlensäurehaltige Limonade
	change of government [ˌtʃeɪndʒ əv 'ɡʌvənmənt]	Regierungswechsel
	to **see an end to sth** [ˌsiː ən 'end tə]	mit etw ein Ende machen
	funding ['fʌndɪŋ]	Finanzierung
	to **apply sth to sth** [ə'plaɪ tə]	etw auf etw anwenden
	to **fail** [feɪl]	scheitern
	to **feed sb** [fiːd]	jdm zu essen geben
	to **be aware about sth** [bi ə'weər əbaʊt]	über etw Bescheid wissen
	to **be considered sth** [bi kən'sɪdəd]	als etw gelten
	posh [pɒʃ]	vornehm, etepetete
	middle class [ˌmɪdl 'klɑːs]	Mittelstand, zum Mittelstand gehörend
	reality [ri'æləti]	Wirklichkeit, Realität
	to **embark on sth** [ɪm'bɑːk ɒn]	etw in Angriff nehmen
	to **rid sth of sth** [rɪd]	etw von etw befreien
	excess ['ekses]	überschüssig
	to **argue** ['ɑːɡjuː]	argumentieren
	effect [ɪ'fekt]	Auswirkung(en), Folge
	extraordinary [ɪk'strɔːdnri]	außerordentlich
	bubble ['bʌbl]	Luftblase
	illegal(ly) [ɪ'liːɡl]	illegal
	pros and cons *pl* [ˌprəʊz ənd 'kɒnz]	Für und Wider

UNIT 8

64	**disorder** [dɪs'ɔːdə]	Störung
	eating disorder [ˌiːtɪŋ dɪs'ɔːdə]	Essstörung
T	**glossy magazine** [ˌɡlɒsi ˌmæɡə'ziːn]	Hochglanzmagazin
	to **accept** [ək'sept]	akzeptieren
	anorexia [ænə'reksiə]	Anorexie
	body weight ['bɒdi weɪt]	Körpergewicht
	bulimia [bjuː'lɪmiə]	Bulimie
	overeating [ˌəʊvər'iːtɪŋ]	übermäßiges Essen
	purging ['pɜːdʒɪŋ]	(kontrolliertes) Erbrechen
	to **overeat** [ˌəʊvər'iːt]	zu viel essen, sich überfressen
	soon enough [ˌsuːn ɪ'nʌf]	früh genug
	to **spot** [spɒt]	erkennen
	to **starve sb/sth of sth** [stɑːv]	jdm/etw etw vorenthalten
	weight loss ['weɪt lɒs]	Gewichtsverlust, -abnahme
	circulation [ˌsɜːkjə'leɪʃn]	Durchblutung, (Blut-) Kreislauf
	enthusiasm [ɪn'θjuːziæzəm]	Begeisterung
	hair loss ['heə lɒs]	Haarausfall
	growth [ɡrəʊθ]	Wachstum, Wuchs
	facial hair ['feɪʃl heə]	Gesichtsbehaarung
	malnutrition [ˌmælnjuː'trɪʃn]	Unterernährung
	bulimic [bjuː'lɪmɪk]	Bulimiker/in
	depressed [dɪ'prest]	deprimiert
	to **purge** [pɜːdʒ]	(kontrolliert) erbrechen
	laxative ['læksətɪv]	Abführmittel
	horrible ['hɒrəbl]	schrecklich, furchtbar
	sufferer ['sʌfərə]	Erkrankte/r, Patient/in
	irregular [ɪ'reɡjələ]	unregelmäßig
	to **deal with sth** ['diːl wɪð]	mit etw fertigwerden, etw bewältigen
	family doctor [ˌfæməli 'dɒktə]	Hausarzt/Hausärztin
	divided by [dɪ'vaɪdɪd baɪ]	geteilt durch
	square [skweə]	Quadrat
	height [haɪt]	Körpergröße
65	to **be sensitive to sth** [bi 'sensətɪv tə]	Verständnis für etw haben, verständnisvoll auf etw reagieren
	emotion [ɪ'məʊʃn]	Gefühl(säußerung), Emotion
	to **encourage** [ɪn'kʌrɪdʒ]	fördern
	ability [ə'bɪləti]	Fähigkeit
	to **ignore** [ɪɡ'nɔː]	ignorieren
	statistics [stə'tɪstɪks]	Statistik(en)
	population [ˌpɒpju'leɪʃn]	Bevölkerung
	to **take steps** [teɪk 'steps]	Schritte unternehmen
	to **address a problem** [əˌres ə 'prɒbləm]	sich mit einem Problem befassen
	facility [fə'sɪləti]	Einrichtung
	generally ['dʒenrəli]	im Allgemeinen
	psychological [ˌsaɪkə'lɒdʒɪkl]	psychologisch
	counselling ['kaʊnsəlɪŋ]	Beratung, Therapie
	nutritional [nju'trɪʃənl]	Ernährungs-
	therapy ['θerəpi]	Therapie
	medical attention [ˌmedɪkl ə'tenʃn]	ärztliche Behandlung, ärztliche Hilfe
	adolescent [ˌædə'lesnt]	heranwachsend, jugendlich
	picky ['pɪki]	wählerisch
	to **miss sth** [mɪs]	etw verpassen
	chance [tʃɑːns]	Gelegenheit, Chance
	to **deal with sth** ['diːl wɪð]	sich mit etw befassen
	to **weigh** [weɪ]	abwiegen, wiegen
	uncontrolled [ˌʌnkən'trəʊld]	unkontrolliert
	dieting ['daɪətɪŋ]	eine Diät machen, Diät(en)
	mood swing ['muːd swɪŋ]	Stimmungsschwankung
	traumatic [trɔː'mætɪk]	traumatisch
	because of sth [bɪ'kɒz əv]	wegen etw
	to **abuse** [ə'bjuːz]	missbrauchen
	failure ['feɪljə]	Scheitern, Versagen
	humiliation [hjuːˌmɪli'eɪʃn]	Demütigung
	to **turn to sth** ['tɜːn tə]	sich einer Sache zuwenden
	in the open [ɪn ði 'əʊpən]	offen
	pushy ['pʊʃi]	aufdringlich, penetrant, aggressiv

	emotional [ɪˈməʊʃənl]	emotional, gefühlsmäßig
	foundation [faʊnˈdeɪʃn]	Fundament
	to **encourage** [ɪnˈkʌrɪdʒ]	ermutigen, ermuntern
	thought [θɔːt]	Gedanke, Überlegung
	to **live up to sth** [ˌlɪv ˈʌp tə]	einer Sache gerecht werden, etw erfüllen
	expectation [ˌekspekˈteɪʃn]	Erwartung
	primarily [praɪˈmerəli]	zu(aller)erst
66	to **populate** [ˈpɒpjuleɪt]	bevölkern
	to **counsel** [ˈkaʊnsl]	beraten
	to **obsess about sth** [əbˈses əbaʊt]	sich andauernd/zwanghaft mit etw beschäftigen
	abuse [əˈbjuːs]	Missbrauch
	to **experience sth** [ɪkˈspɪəriəns]	etw erleben
	unable [ʌnˈeɪbl]	unfähig
	rate [reɪt]	Quote
	childhood [ˈtʃaɪldhʊd]	Kindheit, Jugend
	childhood obesity [ˌtʃaɪldhʊd əʊˈbiːsəti]	Fettleibigkeit bei Kindern und Jugendlichen
	to **triple** [ˈtrɪpl]	sich verdreifachen
	to **reach** [riːtʃ]	erreichen
T	**one in five** [ˌwʌn ɪn ˈfaɪv]	eine/r/s von fünf
	incredible [ɪnˈkredəbl]	unglaublich
	to **hang out with sb** [ˌhæŋ ˈaʊt wɪð]	mit jdm abhängen
	to **copy** [ˈkɒpi]	nachahmen
	surely [ˈʃʊəli]	sicher(lich), bestimmt
	to **play a part in sth** [ˌpleɪ ə ˈpɑːt ɪn]	bei etw eine Rolle spielen
	soccer *AE* [ˈsɒkə]	Fußball
	to **join sb** [dʒɔɪn]	zu jdm gehen, sich zu jdm gesellen
	spending [ˈspendɪŋ]	Ausgaben, Etat
	approximately [əˈprɒksɪmətli]	zirka, ungefähr
	billion [ˈbɪliən]	Milliarde
	to **double** [ˈdʌbl]	sich verdoppeln
67	**journal** [ˈdʒɜːnl]	Zeitschrift
	to **list** [lɪst]	(in einer Liste) aufführen
	sb is sick [ɪz ˈsɪk]	jdm ist schlecht
	mind [maɪnd]	Verstand, Geist, Kopf
	to **act** [ækt]	handeln, sich verhalten
	self-image [ˌself ˈɪmɪdʒ]	Selbstbild
	anorexic [ˌænəˈreksɪk]	Anorektiker/in
	to **starve oneself** [stɑːv]	hungern
	to **binge** [bɪndʒ]	sich vollstopfen
	guilt [gɪlt]	Schuld
	to **meet expectations** [ˌmiːt ekspekˈteɪʃnz]	Erwartungen erfüllen
	power [ˈpaʊə]	Kraft, Macht
	high [haɪ]	Hochgefühl
	to **be in control of sth** [bi ɪn kənˈtrəʊl əv]	etw unter Kontrolle haben
	binge [bɪndʒ]	Fressattacke
	purge [pɜːdʒ]	(kontrolliertes) Erbrechen
	to **fight sb** [faɪt]	jdn bekämpfen, gegen jnd kämpfen
	motivation [ˌməʊtɪˈveɪʃn]	Motivation
	hopelessness [ˈhəʊpləsnəs]	Hoffnungslosigkeit
	to **take your life** [ˌteɪk jɔː ˈlaɪf]	sich umbringen
68	**guilty** [ˈgɪlti]	schuldig
	unit [ˈjuːnɪt]	Einheit, Maßeinheit
	everyday [ˈevrideɪ]	Alltags-, alltäglich
	consumption [kənˈsʌmpʃn]	Verzehr, Konsum, Verbrauch
	usage [ˈjuːsɪdʒ]	Verbrauch
	to **raise** [reɪz]	erhöhen
	clause [klɔːz]	Satzglied, Nebensatz
	to **respond to sth** [rɪˈspɒnd tə]	auf etw reagieren, auf etw *(Behandlung usw.)* ansprechen
	to **take sth seriously** [teɪk ˈsɪəriəsli]	etw ernst nehmen
	unfortunately [ʌnˈfɔːtʃənətli]	leider
	research [rɪˈsɜːtʃ]	Recherche, Nachforschungen
	to **research sth** [rɪˈsɜːtʃ]	etw recherchieren, Nachforschungen über etw anstellen
	fried egg [fraɪd ˈeg]	Spiegelei
	boiled [bɔɪld]	gekocht
	whole milk [ˌhəʊl ˈmɪlk]	Vollmilch
	peanut butter [ˈpiːnʌt bʌtə]	Erdnussbutter
	apricot [ˈeɪprɪkɒt]	Aprikose
70	**slim** [slɪm]	schlank
	mixed up [ˌmɪkst ˈʌp]	durcheinander, vertauscht
	catwalk [ˈkætwɔːk]	Laufsteg
	presenter [prɪˈzentə]	Moderator/in
	diet [ˈdaɪət]	Diät
	tummy [ˈtʌmi]	Bauch
	flat [flæt]	flach
	even though [ˈiːvn ðəʊ]	obwohl
	excited [ɪkˈsaɪtɪd]	aufgeregt, freudig erregt
	to **cut back** [ˌkʌt ˈbæk]	kürzen, zurückschrauben
	madness [ˈmædnəs]	Irrsinn
	starvation [stɑːˈveɪʃn]	Hungern, Unterernährung
	challenge [ˈtʃælɪndʒ]	Herausforderung, Kampfansage, Wettstreit
	comfort [ˈkʌmfət]	Trost
	permanent [ˈpɜːmənənt]	dauernd
	mineral levels *pl* [ˈmɪnərəl levlz]	Mineralstoffgehalt
	period [ˈpɪəriəd]	Periode
	to **risk** [rɪsk]	riskieren, Gefahr laufen
	to **grow** [grəʊ]	wachsen, werden
	constipation [ˌkɒnstɪˈpeɪʃn]	Verstopfung
	immune system [ɪˈmjuːn sɪstəm]	Immunsystem
	dress size [ˈdres saɪz]	Kleidergröße
	unattractive [əˌʌnˈtræktɪv]	unattraktiv
	Uruguayan [ˌjʊrəˈgwaɪən]	aus Uruguay

	lettuce leaves *pl* [ˈletɪs liːvz]	Salatblätter
	World Health Organization (WHO) [ˌwɜːld ˈhelθ ɔːgənaɪzeɪʃn]	Weltgesundheitsorganisation
	to consider sth to be [kənˈsɪdə]	etw für etw halten
	joy (of sth) [dʒɔɪ]	Freude (über etw)
	to kick in [ˌkɪk ˈɪn]	einsetzen
	for no reason [fə nəʊ ˈriːzn]	ohne Grund
	insecure [ˌɪnsɪˈkjʊə]	unsicher, verunsichert
	disaster [dɪˈzɑːstə]	Katastrophe
	jealous (of sth) [ˈdʒeləs]	eifersüchtig (auf etw), neidisch (auf etw)
	thinness [ˈθɪnnəs]	Schlankheit
	crash diet [ˌkræʃ ˈdaɪət]	Radikalkur, Radikaldiät
	crew [kruː]	Team
	to record [rɪˈkɔːd]	aufnehmen, *hier:* filmen
	curvy [ˈkɜːvi]	kurvig
	skinny [ˈskɪni]	mager, dürr
	aim [eɪm]	Ziel, Absicht
	miserable [ˈmɪzrəbl]	elend
71	**to feature** [ˈfiːtʃə]	*(in einer Zeitschrift)* bringen
	unnatural(ly) [ʌnˈnætʃrəl]	unnatürlich
	constant(ly) [ˈkɒnstənt]	ständig
	to produce [prəˈdjuːs]	erstellen, herstellen
	tip [tɪp]	Hinweis, Tipp

UNIT 9

72	**to screen sb for sth** [ˈskriːn fə]	jdn auf etw hin untersuchen
	screening [ˈskriːnɪŋ]	Untersuchung *(auf etw Bestimmtes)*
T	**lump** [lʌmp]	Knoten
T	**to make a fuss** [ˌmeɪk ə ˈfʌs]	sich anstellen, Theater machen
T	**suspicious** [səˈspɪʃəs]	verdächtig
T	**mammogram** [ˈmæməgræm]	Mammographie
T	**cycle** [ˈsaɪkl]	Zyklus
T	**to breast-feed** [ˈbrest fiːd]	stillen
	force [fɔːs]	Kraft
	unimportant [ˌʌnɪmˈpɔːtənt]	unwichtig, unbedeutend
	ovulation [ˌɒvjuːˈleɪ.ʃən]	Eisprung, Ovulation
	menstruation [ˌmenstruˈeɪʃn]	Menstruation
	solid [ˈsɒlɪd]	fest, hart
	specific [spəˈsɪfɪk]	konkret, genau
	shape [ʃeɪp]	Form
	automatic(ally) [ˌɔːtəˈmætɪk]	automatisch
	to invite [ɪnˈvaɪt]	einladen
	specialist [ˈspeʃəlɪst]	Fach-, Spezial-
	society [səˈsaɪəti]	Gesellschaft
	unit [ˈjuːnɪt]	Gerät
	radiology [ˌreɪdiˈɒlədʒi]	Radiologie
73	**area** [ˈeəriə]	Bereich
	to remove [rɪˈmuːv]	entfernen, *(Kleidung)* ablegen
	upper clothing [ˌʌpə ˈkləʊðɪŋ]	Oberbekleidung
	bra [brɑː]	BH
	screen [skriːn]	Trennwand, Vorhang
	privacy [ˈprɪvəsi]	Privatsphäre
	to get undressed [ˌget ʌnˈdrest]	sich ausziehen
	armpit [ˈɑːmpɪt]	Achselhöhle
	to raise [reɪz]	hochheben
	gentle [ˈdʒentl]	sanft
	to press [pres]	drücken
	cyst [sɪst]	Zyste
	ultrasound [ˈʌltrəsaʊnd]	Ultraschall
	examination table [ɪgˌzæmɪˈneɪʃn teɪbl]	Untersuchungsliege
	machine [məˈʃiːn]	Gerät
	instruction(s) [ɪnˈstrʌkʃn]	Aufforderung
	helpful [ˈhelpfl]	hilfreich, nützlich
74	**acoustic gel** [əˌkuːstɪk ˈdʒel]	Ultraschallgel
	pillow [ˈpɪləʊ]	Kopfkissen
T	**to mark sth** [mɑːk]	auf etw Flecken hinterlassen
T	**at first** [ət ˈfɜːst]	zunächst
T	**to turn** [tɜːn]	(sich) wenden
T	**outside** [ˈaʊtsaɪd]	Außenseite
T	**to panic** [ˈpænɪk]	in Panik geraten
T	**there's no point in doing sth** [ðeəz ˌnəʊ ˈpɔɪnt ɪn duːɪŋ]	es hat keinen Sinn, etw zu tun
T	**benign** [bɪˈnaɪn]	gutartig
T	**malignant** [məˈlɪgnənt]	bösartig
T	**tumour** [ˈtjuːmə]	Geschwulst, Tumor
T	**recovery** [rɪˈkʌvəri]	Genesung
T	**to get dressed** [get ˈdrest]	sich anziehen
T	**for sure** [fə ˈʃʊə]	(ganz) sicher
75	**issue** [ˈɪʃuː]	Problem
	training session [ˈtreɪnɪŋ seʃn]	Fortbildung, Lehrgang
	alcohol [ˈælkəhɒl]	Alkohol
	presenter [prɪˈzentə]	Vortragende/r, Dozent/in
	flow chart [ˈfləʊ tʃɑːt]	Flussdiagramm
T	**handout** [ˈhændaʊt]	Arbeitsblatt, Informationsblatt
T	**to interact with sth** [ˌɪntərˈækt wɪð]	eine Wechselwirkung mit etw haben
T	**high-risk patient** [haɪ ˌrɪsk ˈpeɪʃnt]	Risikopatient
T	**adolescent** [ˌædəˈlesnt]	Heranwachsende/r
T	**related** [rɪˈleɪtɪd]	bezogen
T	**liver** [ˈlɪvə]	Leber

	prescreen [ˈpriːskriːn]	Voruntersuchung, Vorgespräch
	questionnaire [ˌkwestʃəˈneə]	Fragebogen
	to **hand sth out** [ˌhænd ˈaʊt]	etw austeilen
	copy [ˈkɒpi]	Exemplar
	heavy [ˈhevi]	schwer
	to **remind sb of sth** [rɪˈmaɪnd]	jdn an etw erinnern
	limit [ˈlɪmɪt]	Höchstgrenze, Grenzwert
	to **assess (sb for sth)** [əˈses]	(jdn in Hinsicht auf etw) beurteilen, bewerten, einschätzen
	alcohol-use disorder [ˌælkəhɒl juːs dɪsˈɔːdə]	alkoholbezogene Störung
	to **concern** [kənˈsɜːn]	betreffen
	dependence [dɪˈpendəns]	Abhängigkeit
	to **agree sth** [əˈgriː]	sich auf etw einigen
	goal [gəʊl]	Ziel
	follow-up [ˈfɒləʊ ʌp]	Folge-
	to **stress** [stres]	betonen
	to **continue sth** [kənˈtɪnjuː]	mit etw weitermachen
	final [ˈfaɪnl]	letzte/r/s
	support group [səˈpɔːt gruːp]	Selbsthilfegruppe
	Alcoholics Anonymous [ælkəˌhɒlɪks əˈnɒnɪməs]	Anonyme Alkoholiker
	possibility [ˌpɒsəˈbɪləti]	Möglichkeit
	complete [kəmˈpliːt]	abgeschlossen
	to **brainstorm** [ˈbreɪnstɔːm]	Ideen sammeln
	to **define** [dɪˈfaɪn]	definieren
76	**under-age** [ˌʌndərˈeɪdʒ]	minderjährig, bei/von Minderjährigen
	minimum [ˈmɪnɪməm]	Mindest-, mindestens
	minimum legal age [ˌmɪnɪməm ˌliːgl ˈeɪdʒ]	gesetzliches Mindestalter
	drug [drʌg]	Droge
	to **experiment** [ɪkˈsperɪmənt]	experimentieren
	to **consume** [kənˈsjuːm]	konsumieren
	period of time [ˈpɪəriəd əv taɪm]	Zeitspanne
	to **down** [daʊn]	*(Getränk)* hinunterkippen
	in a row [ɪn ə ˈrəʊ]	nacheinander
	peer pressure [ˈpɪə preʃə]	Gruppendruck/-zwang
	sip [sɪp]	(kleiner) Schluck
	to **binge** [bɪndʒ]	sich vollsaufen
	to **keep up** [ˌkiːp ˈʌp]	Schritt halten
	to **circulate** [ˈsɜːkjəleɪt]	zirkulieren, fließen
	bloodstream [ˈblʌdstriːm]	Blutkreislauf
	drunk [drʌŋk]	betrunken
	for instance [fəˈrɪnstəns]	zum Beispiel
	fatal [ˈfeɪtl]	tödlich
	car crash [ˈkɑː kræʃ]	Autounfall
	wheel [wiːl]	Rad, *hier:* Lenkrad, Steuer
	to begin with [tə bɪˈgɪn wɪð]	zunächst (einmal)
	to **fall behind** [ˌfɔːl bɪˈhaɪnd]	zurückfallen
	to **injure** [ˈɪndʒə]	verletzen
	to **damage** [ˈdæmɪdʒ]	beschädigen
	property [ˈprɒpəti]	Eigentum
	increased [ɪnˈkriːst]	erhöht
	sexually transmitted disease (STD) [ˌsekʃuəli trænsˌmɪtɪd dɪˈziːz]	sexuell übertragbare Krankheit
	to **delay** [dɪˈleɪ]	verzögern
	puberty [ˈpjuːbəti]	Pubertät
	to **hurt** [hɜːt]	verletzen
	so-called [ˌsəʊˈkɔːld]	sogenannt
	grey matter [ˌgreɪ ˈmætə]	die grauen Zellen
	region [ˈriːdʒən]	Bereich, Region
	prefrontal cortex [priːˌfrɒntəl ˈkɔːteks]	präfrontale Cortex
	attention [əˈtenʃn]	Aufmerksamkeit
	self-control [ˌself kənˈtrəʊl]	Selbstbeherrschung
	decision [dɪˈsɪʒn]	Entscheidung
	to **make a decision** [ˌmeɪk ə dɪˈsɪʒn]	eine Entscheidung fällen
	to **turn sth down** [ˌtɜːn ˈdaʊn]	etw ablehnen
	inappropriate [ˌɪnəˈprəʊpriət]	unangemessen
	behaviour [bɪˈheɪvjə]	Verhalten, Benehmen
	alcoholism [ˈælkəhɒlɪzəm]	Alkoholismus, Alkoholsucht
77	**longer-term** [ˌlɒŋgə ˈtɜːm]	längerfristig
	according to [əˈkɔːdɪŋ tə]	laut, nach, gemäß
	author [ˈɔːθə]	Autor/in, Verfasser/in
	to **specify** [ˈspesɪfaɪ]	genau angeben
	to **slow sth down** [ˌsləʊ ˈdaʊn]	etw bremsen, etw verzögern
	progress [ˈprəʊgres]	Fortgang, Fortschreiten
79	**since** [sɪns]	da, weil
	drug user [ˈdrʌg juːzə]	Drogenabhängige/r
	synthetic [sɪnˈθetɪk]	synthetisch
	cannabinoid [ˈkænəbɪnɔɪd]	Cannabinoid
	similar (to sth) [ˈsɪmələ]	(einer Sache) ähnlich
	dissimilar (to sth) [dɪˈsɪmɪlə]	(von etw) verschieden
	deadly [ˈdedli]	tödlich
	chemist [ˈkemɪst]	Chemiker/in
	purpose [ˈpɜːpəs]	Zweck
	to **imagine** [ɪˈmædʒɪn]	sich (etw) vorstellen
	recreational [ˌrekriˈeɪʃənl]	Erholungs-, Freizeit-
	powerful [ˈpaʊəfl]	stark
	marijuana [ˌmærəˈwɑːnə]	Marihuana
	to **spray** [spreɪ]	sprühen
	plant [plɑːnt]	Pflanze
	huge [hjuːdʒ]	riesengroß, riesig
	range [reɪndʒ]	Reihe, Spektrum

since [sɪns]	seit
to **appear** [əˈpɪə]	erscheinen
initials *pl* [ɪˈnɪʃlz]	Initialen
set [set]	Menge
agitation [ˌædʒɪˈteɪʃn]	Unruhe, Erregung
vomiting [ˈvɒmɪtɪŋ]	Erbrechen
hallucination [həˌluːsɪˈneɪʃn]	Wahnvorstellung(en), Halluzination(en)
paranoia [ˌpærəˈnɔɪə]	Verfolgungswahn, Paranoia
seizure [ˈsiːʒə]	(epileptischer) Anfall
stroke [strəʊk]	Schlaganfall
kidney [ˈkɪdni]	Niere
acute [əˈkjuːt]	akut
psychosis [saɪˈkəʊsɪs]	Psychose
ingredient [ɪnˈgriːdiənt]	Bestandteil
tetrahydrocannabinol (THC) [ˌtetrəhaɪdrəʊkəˈnæbɪnɒl]	Tetrahydrocannabinol (THC)
to **act on sth** [ˈækt ɒn]	auf etw wirken
receptor [rɪˈseptə]	Rezeptor
central nervous system [ˌsentrəl ˌnɜːvəs ˈsɪstəm]	Zentrales Nervensystem
to **activate** [ˈæktɪveɪt]	aktivieren
endocannabinoid [ˌendəʊˈkænəbɪnɔɪd]	Endocannabinoid
long-lasting [ˌlɒŋ ˈlɑːstɪŋ]	dauerhaft
compound [ˈkɒmpaʊnd]	(chemische) Verbindung
to **affect sth** [əˈfekt]	sich auf etw auswirken
severe [sɪˈvɪə]	heftig, schlimm, schwer
proof [pruːf]	Beweis(e)
overdose [ˈəʊvədəʊs]	Überdosis
in no way [ɪn ˌnəʊ ˈweɪ]	in keiner Weise
to **tend to do sth** [ˈtend tə]	dazu neigen, etw zu tun
interactive [ˌɪntərˈæktɪv]	kommunikativ
on the other hand [ɒn ði ˈʌðə hænd]	andererseits
agitated [ˈedʒɪteɪtɪd]	unruhig, aufgeregt
to **sweat profusely** [ˌswet prəˈfjuːsli]	stark schwitzen
regulation [ˌregjuˈleɪʃn]	Gesetzgebung, Vorschriften
not particularly [ˌnɒt pəˈtɪkjələli]	nicht besonders
graduate [ˈgrædʒuət]	Absolvent/in
chemistry [ˈkemɪstri]	Chemie
secret [ˈsiːkrɪt]	geheim
in the lead [ɪn ðə ˈliːd]	ganz vorn
production [prəˈdʌkʃn]	Herstellung, Produktion
to **impose sth** [ɪmˈpəʊz]	etw durchsetzen
quality control [ˈkwɒləti kəntrəʊl]	Qualitätskontrolle
authorities *pl* [ɔːˈθɒrətiz]	Behörden
as soon as [əz ˈsuːn əz]	sobald
to **manage** [ˈmænɪdʒ]	(es) schaffen
producer [prəˈdjuːsə]	Hersteller/in, Produzent/in

UNIT 10

80	to **apply to sb for sth** [əˈplaɪ]	sich bei jdm um etw bewerben
	characteristic [ˌkærəktəˈrɪstɪk]	Merkmal, Kennzeichen
	senior [ˈsiːniə]	leitend, vorgesetzt, ranghöher
	general practice nurse *BE* [ˌdʒenrəl ˈpræktɪs nɜːs]	*brit. Arzthelfer/in, die ausschließlich Behandlungsaufgaben erledigt*
	reliable [rɪˈlaɪəbl]	zuverlässig
	confident [ˈkɒnfɪdənt]	selbstbewusst
	talkative [ˈtɔːkətɪv]	gesprächig
	cheerful [ˈtʃɪəfl]	gut gelaunt, fröhlich
	listener [ˈlɪsnə]	Zuhörer/in
	well-organized [ˌwelˈɔːgənaɪzd]	gut organisiert
	highly qualified [ˌhaɪli ˈkwɒlɪfaɪd]	hochqualifiziert
	responsible [rɪˈspɒnsəbl]	verantwortungsbewusst
	accurate [ˈækjərət]	genau, akkurat
	vocational qualification [vəʊˌkeɪʃənl kwɒlɪfɪˈkeɪʃn]	Berufsabschluss
	certified [ˈsɜːtɪfaɪd]	(staatlich) geprüft
	nursing assistant [ˈnɜːsɪŋ əsɪstənt]	Pflegehelfer/in
	vocational course [vəʊˌkeɪʃənl ˈkɔːs]	Berufsbildungskurs
	licensed practical nurse *AE* [ˌlaɪsnst ˌpræktɪkl ˈnɜːs]	staatlich geprüfte/r Krankenpflegehelfer/in
	community college *AE* [kəˈmjuːnəti kɒlɪdʒ]	*weiterbildende und Berufsschule in den USA, die auch Erwachsenen offensteht*
	vocational school [vəʊˌkeɪʃənl ˈskuːl]	Berufsschule
	registered nurse [ˌredʒɪstəd ˈnɜːs]	examinierte/r Krankenschwester/-pfleger
	level [ˈlevl]	Stufe, Ebene
	university [ˌjuːnɪˈvɜːsəti]	Universität
81	**apprenticeship** [əˈprentɪʃɪp]	Ausbildung, Lehre
	to **approve** [əˈpruːv]	anerkennen
	nursing [ˈnɜːsɪŋ]	Krankenpflege
	midwifery [ˌmɪdˈwɪfəri]	Geburtshilfe
	council [ˈkaʊnsl]	Rat
	membership [ˈmembəʃɪp]	Mitgliedschaft
	membership organization [ˈmembəʃɪp ɔːgənaɪzeɪʃn]	Fachverband, Berufsverband
	job advertisment [ˈdʒɒb ədvɜːtɪsmənt]	Stellenanzeige, -ausschreibung
	advert(isment) [ˈædvɜːt]	Anzeige
	requirement [rɪˈkwaɪəmənt]	Anforderung
	work routine [ˌwɜːk ruːˈtiːn]	Arbeitsablauf

	organizational [ˌɔːɡənaɪˈzeɪʃənl]	organisatorisch, Organisations-
	experienced [ɪkˈspɪəriənst]	erfahren
	staff nurse [ˌstɑːf ˈnɜːs]	examinierte/r Krankenschwester/-pfleger
	assessment [əˈsesmənt]	Einschätzung, Beurteilung
	assessment skills *pl* [əˈsesmənt skɪlz]	Einschätzungsvermögen
	decision-making [dɪˈsɪʒn meɪkɪŋ]	Entscheidungsfindung
	range [reɪndʒ]	Reihe, Auswahl
	verbal [ˈvɜːbl]	mündlich
	desirable [dɪˈzaɪərəbl]	erwünscht
	evidence [ˈevɪdəns]	Nachweis
	care assistant [ˌkeər əˈsɪstənt]	Pflegeassistent/in
	oak [əʊk]	Eiche
	retirement [rɪˈtaɪəmənt]	Ruhestand
	to **require** [rɪˈkwaɪə]	benötigen
	interpersonal skills *pl* [ˌɪntəˈpɜːsənl skɪlz]	soziale Kompetenz
	elderly people [ˌeldəli ˈpiːpl]	ältere Menschen, Senioren
	smart [smɑːt]	intelligent, aufgeweckt
	enthusiastic about sth [ɪnˌθjuːziˈæstɪk əbaʊt]	von etw begeistert
	to **care for sb** [ˈkeə fə]	jdn betreuen, sich um jdn kümmern, jdn pflegen
	in writing [ɪn ˈraɪtɪŋ]	schriftlich
	nursing home [ˈnɜːsɪŋ həʊm]	Pflegeheim
	to **handle** [ˈhændl]	erledigen
	inquiry [ɪnˈkwaɪəri]	Anfrage
	to **be designed to do sth** [bi dɪˈzaɪnd tə]	dafür gedacht sein, etw zu tun
	paperless [ˈpeɪpələs]	papierfrei
82	**as well as** [əz ˈwel əz]	ebenso wie
	previous [ˈpriːviəs]	vorige/r/s
T	**… and stuff** [ənd ˈstʌf]	… und so
	to **make use of sth** [ˌmeɪk ˈjuːs əv]	etw nutzen, sich etw zunutze machen
	career [kəˈrɪə]	Beruf, Laufbahn, Karriere
	to **mind** [maɪnd]	etw dagegen haben
	temping agency [ˈtempɪŋ eɪdʒənsi]	Zeitarbeitsfirma
	temporary [ˈtemprəri]	befristet
	secretarial [ˌsekrəˈteəriəl]	Sekretariats-
	application [ˌæplɪˈkeɪʃn]	Bewerbung
	letter of application [ˌletər əv æplɪˈkeɪʃn]	Bewerbungsschreiben
	to **advertise** [ˈædvətaɪz]	*(Stelle)* ausschreiben
	shop assistant [ˈʃɒp əsɪstənt]	Verkäufer/in
	department store [dɪˈpɑːtmənt stɔː]	Kaufhaus
	sales target [ˈseɪlz tɑːɡɪt]	Umsatzziel, Verkaufsziel
	enclosed [ɪnˈkləʊzd]	*(Brief:)* beigefügt
	curriculum vitae (CV) [kəˌrɪkjələm ˈviːtaɪ]	Lebenslauf
	to **marry** [ˈmæri]	heiraten
	advertisment [ədˈvɜːtɪsmənt]	Anzeige, Annonce
	to **be available for sth** [bi əˈveɪləbl fə]	für etw zur Verfügung stehen
	to **look forward to sth** [ˌlʊk ˈfɔːwəd tə]	sich auf etw freuen
	Yours sincerely [ˌjɔːz sɪnˈsɪəli]	*(Brief:)* Mit freundlichen Grüßen
	enc(losures *pl***)** [ɪnˈkləʊʒəz]	*(Brief:)* Anlagen
	currently [ˈkʌrəntli]	derzeit, zurzeit, momentan
83	to **rest with sth** [ˈrest wɪð]	auf etw ruhen
	career ladder [kəˈrɪə lædə]	Karriereleiter
	to **represent** [ˌreprɪˈzent]	darstellen
	to **miss out on sth** [ˌmɪs ˈaʊt ɒn]	sich etw entgehen lassen
	to **attract sb's attention** [əˌtrækt əˈtenʃn]	jds Aufmerksamkeit fesseln
	employer [ɪmˈplɔɪə]	Arbeitgeber/in
	section break [ˈsekʃn breɪk]	Abschnittswechsel
	hand-written [ˌhændˈrɪtn]	handgeschrieben
	old-fashioned [ˌəʊldˈfæʃənd]	altmodisch
	out of date [ˌaʊt əv ˈdeɪt]	veraltet
	life history [ˌlaɪf ˈhɪstri]	Lebensgeschichte
	mobile phone [ˌməʊbaɪl ˈfəʊn]	Mobiltelefon
	marital status [ˌmærɪtl ˈsteɪtəs]	Familienstand
	nationality [ˌnæʃəˈnæləti]	Staatsangehörigkeit
	abroad [əˈbrɔːd]	im Ausland
	a must [ə ˈmʌst]	ein Muss
	professional association [prəˌfeʃənl əsəʊsiˈeɪʃn]	Berufsverband
	to **complete sth** [kəmˈpliːt]	etw *(Studium usw.)* abschließen
	subject [ˈsʌbdʒɪkt]	(Schul-, Studien-)Fach
	relevant to [ˈreləvənt tə]	relevant für, wichtig für
	backwards [ˈbækwədz]	rückwärts
	to **set out sth** [ˌset ˈaʊt]	etw darlegen
	responsibility [rɪˌspɒnsəˈbɪləti]	Verantwortlichkeit, Zuständigkeit
	achievement [əˈtʃiːvmənt]	Leistung, Errungenschaft, Erfolg
	to **transfer** [trænsˈfɜː]	übertragen
	foreign language skills *pl* [ˌfɒrən ˈlæŋɡwɪdʒ skɪlz]	Fremdsprachenkenntnisse
	to **indicate** [ˈɪndɪkeɪt]	angeben
	technical [ˈteknɪkl]	technisch, Fach-
	strength [streŋθ]	Stärke
	versatile [ˈvɜːsətaɪl]	vielseitig
	motivate [ˈməʊtɪveɪt]	motivieren

	staff appraisal ['stɑ:f əpreɪzl]	Mitarbeiterbeurteilung
	reference ['refərəns]	Referenz, Zeugnis
	surprising [sə'praɪzɪŋ]	erstaunlich
84	**comprehensive school** [kɒmprɪ'hensɪv sku:l]	Gesamtschule
	equivalent [ɪ'kwɪvələnt]	Entsprechung
	sales area [ˌseɪlz 'eəriə]	Verkaufsfläche
	stock levels *pl* ['stɒk levlz]	Lagerbestände
	sandwich release ['sænwɪdʒ rɪli:s]	blockweise Freistellung
	native speaker [ˌneɪtɪv 'spi:kə]	Muttersprachler/in
	good command [ˌgʊd kə'mɑ:nd]	gute Beherrschung
	intermediate French [ɪntəˌmi:diət 'frentʃ]	Französisch auf fortgeschrittenem Anfängerniveau
	driving licence ['draɪvɪŋ laɪsns]	Führerschein
85	to **attach** [ə'tætʃ]	*(Brief:)* beifügen
	prompt [prɒmpt]	Stichwort
86	**careers adviser** [kə'rɪəz ədvaɪzə]	Berufsberater/in
	employment agency [ɪm'plɔɪmənt eɪdʒənsi]	Arbeitsvermittlung
T	**stressful** ['stresfl]	anstrengend, stressig
	preparation [ˌprepə'reɪʃn]	Vorbereitung
	beforehand [bɪ'fɔ:hænd]	vorher
	traffic ['træfɪk]	(Straßen-)Verkehr
	sensible ['sensəbl]	vernünftig
	to **match sth to sth** [mætʃ]	etw an etw anpassen
	to **sound** [saʊnd]	klingen
	Practice makes perfect. [ˌpræktɪs meɪks 'pɜ:fɪkt]	Übung macht den Meister.
	appearance [ə'pɪərəns]	(äußere) Erscheinung, Erscheinungsbild
	smart [smɑ:t]	*(Kleidung:)* schick
	jewellery ['dʒu:əlri]	Schmuck
	in advance [ɪn əd'vɑ:ns]	im Voraus
	relaxing bath [rɪˌlæksɪŋ 'bɑ:θ]	Entspannungsbad
	to **make friends** [meɪk 'frendz]	Freunde finden
	to **stay awake** [ˌsteɪ ə'weɪk]	wach bleiben
	skydiving ['skaɪdaɪvɪŋ]	Fallschirmspringen
	employee [ɪm'plɔɪi:]	Angestellte/r
	interviewer ['ɪntəvju:ə]	jd, der ein Vorstellungsgespräch führt
	interviewee [ˌɪntəvju:'i:]	Befragte/r, Bewerber(in)
	trainer ['treɪnə]	Ausbilder/in
	role-play ['rəʊl pleɪ]	Rollenspiel
88	**pub** [pʌb]	Kneipe
	retail ['ri:teɪl]	Einzelhandel
	nerve-racking ['nɜ:v rækɪŋ]	nervenaufreibend
	broad [brɔ:d]	breit
	pay [peɪ]	Bezahlung
	future ['fju:tʃə]	zukünftig, für die Zukunft
	to **qualify** ['kwɒlɪfaɪ]	den Abschluss machen

AZ A–Z word list

Diese Liste enthält alle Wörter der Units 1–10 in alphabetischer Reihenfolge (ohne Grundwortschatz – siehe *Basic word list*). T = Das Wort befindet sich im Transkript der Hörverständnistexte.

A

A & E (department) *23T* Notaufnahme
ability *65* Fähigkeit
abroad *83* im Ausland
absolutely *51T* völlig, absolut, ganz
abuse *66* Missbrauch
to **abuse** *65* missbrauchen
to **accept** *64T* akzeptieren
acceptable *11* akzeptabel
accident *14* Unfall
according to *77* laut, nach, gemäß
to **account for sth** *60* etw ausmachen
accounting *13* Buchführung
accounts *pl* *7* Buchhaltung
accuracy *43* Genauigkeit
accurate *80* genau, akkurat
to **ache** *33* schmerzen
to **achieve** *12* erreichen, erlangen
achievement *83* Leistung, Errungenschaft, Erfolg
acid, folic ~ *57T* Folsäure
acoustic gel *74* Ultraschallgel
across … *45* im gesamten …; **~ sth** *45* auf der anderen Seite von etw
to **act** *67* handeln, sich verhalten; **~ on sth** *79* auf etw wirken
action *23* Handlung, Maßnahme, Aktion; to **take ~** *23* Maßnahme(n) ergreifen
to **activate** *79* aktivieren
activity *32* Tätigkeit, Aktivität
actual *41* wirklich, tatsächlich
actually *27* wirklich, eigentlich, tatsächlich
acute *79* akut
addition, in ~ to sth *13* zusätzlich zu etw
additional *37* zusätzlich, Zusatz-
to **address a problem** *65* sich mit einem Problem befassen
administration *7* Verwaltung
administrator, medical ~ *12* Arzthelfer/in (für Verwaltungsaufgaben)
adolescent *65* heranwachsend, jugendlich; *75T* Heranwachsende/r
advance, in ~ *86T* im Voraus
advantage *45* Vorteil, Vorzug
advert(isment) *81* Anzeige, Annonce; **job ~** *81* Stellenanzeige, -ausschreibung
to **advertise** *82* *(Stelle)* ausschreiben
advice *21* Beratung, Rat
to **advise** *59* raten, beraten
adviser *78* Berater/in; **careers ~** *86* Berufsberater/in
to **affect** *12* beeinflussen; *37* betreffen; **~ sth** *79* sich auf etw auswirken
afraid, I'm ~ *10T* leider; to **be ~ of sb/sth** *47* sich vor jdm/etw fürchten
age, minimum legal ~ *76* gesetzliches Mindestalter
aged *42* im Alter von
agency *78* Agentur; **employment ~** *86* Arbeitsvermittlung; **temping ~** *82T* Zeitarbeitsfirma
agitated *79* unruhig, aufgeregt
agitation *79* Unruhe, Erregung
to **agree** *34* zustimmen; **~ sth** *75T* sich auf etw einigen
aid, first ~ *13* Erste Hilfe; **hearing ~** *47* Hörgerät
aim *70* Ziel, Absicht
air *32T* Luft
alcohol *75* Alkohol; **~-use disorder** *75T* alkoholbezogene Störung
Alcoholics Anonymous *75T* Anonyme Alkoholiker
alcoholism *76* Alkoholismus, Alkoholsucht
all, at ~ *31* überhaupt
allergic (to sth) *29T* allergisch (gegen etw)
to **allow** *17* gestatten, erlauben; **~ sth for sth** *43* etw für etw vorsehen; **~ to dissolve** *52* zergehen lassen
almost *42* fast, beinah
alternative(ly) *21* alternativ
although *24* obwohl
ambulance *37* Rettungswagen
amount *57* Menge
anaesthetic *29T* Betäubungsmittel; to **give local ~** *39* örtlich betäuben
analyis *78* Analyse
to **analyse** *7* untersuchen, analysieren
anatomy *13* Anatomie
angry *55T* ungehalten, wütend
animal *57T* tierisch
anorexia *64T* Anorexie
anorexic *67* Anorektiker/in
antibiotic *23T* Antibiotikum
anxiety *47* Angst, Ängstlichkeit, Besorgnis
anxious *7* ängstlich, besorgt, nervös; to **be ~ about sth** *47* sich um/wegen etw Sorgen machen
any more, not … ~ *9* nicht mehr
anyway *32T* also, wie dem auch sei
to **apologize** *55T* sich entschuldigen
to **appear** *79* erscheinen
appearance *86T* (äußere) Erscheinung, Erscheinungsbild
applicant *13* Bewerber/in
application *82* Bewerbung; **letter of ~** *82* Bewerbungsschreiben
to **apply** *11* *(Make-up)* auftragen; **~ for sth** *31* sich um etw bewerben; **~ to sb** *44* auf jdn zutreffen; **~ sth to sth** *63* etw auf etw anwenden; **~ to sb for sth** *80* sich bei jdm um etw bewerben
appointment *6* Termin; **~ book** *15* Terminkalender; **~ card** *26* Terminkarte; **electronic ~ book** *26* elektronischer Terminkalender
appraisal, staff ~ *83* Mitarbeiterbeurteilung
apprenticeship *81* Ausbildung, Lehre
appropriateness *11* Angemessenheit, Schicklichkeit
to **approve** *81* anerkennen; **~ sth** *44* etw zulassen
approximately *66* zirka, ungefähr
apricot *68* Aprikose
area *73* Bereich
to **argue** *63* argumentieren
armpit *73* Achselhöhle
aromatherapy *49* Aromatherapie
artery *42* Arterie; **brachial ~** *43* Oberarmarterie
article *37* Artikel
as: ~ far as *33* soweit; **~ if** *45* als ob; **~ soon as** *79* sobald; **~ well** *34T* auch, und; **~ well as** *82* ebenso wie
to **ask for directions** *25* nach dem Weg fragen
aspect *13* Gesichtspunkt, Seite, Aspekt
to **assess (sb for sth)** *75T* (jdn in Hinsicht auf etw) beurteilen, bewerten, einschätzen
assessment *81* Einschätzung, Beurteilung; **~ skills** *pl* *81* Einschätzungsvermögen
assignment *12* Aufgabe; **work-based ~** *12* praktische Prüfungsaufgabe
to **assist** *13* helfen, unterstützen; **~ sb** *6* jdm assistieren
assistance *17* Hilfe, Unterstützung

assistant *6* Assistent/in, Helfer/in; **care ~** *81* Pflegeassistent/in; **medical ~** *6* Medizinische Fachangestellte/r; **nursing ~** *80* Pflegehelfer/in; **shop ~** *82* Verkäufer/in

assisting, clinical ~ *AE 13* Behandlungsassistenz

associate degree *AE 13 US-Abschluss, der nach zwei Jahren verliehen wird*

to **associate sb with sth** *48* jdn mit etw in Verbindung bringen

association *12* Verband, Vereinigung; **professional ~** *83* Berufsverband

asthma *30* Asthma

athletic shoes *pl 11* Sportschuhe

atmosphere *48* Atmosphäre, Stimmung

to **attach** *26* zusammenfügen; *85 (Brief:)* beifügen; **~ to sth** *44* sich an etw (fest)setzen

attack, heart ~ *37* Herzinfarkt

attention *76* Aufmerksamkeit; to **attract sb's ~** *83* jds Aufmerksamkeit fesseln; to **pay ~ to sth** *61* auf etw achten; **medical ~** *65* ärztliche Behandlung, ärztliche Hilfe

to **attract sb's attention** *83* jds Aufmerksamkeit fesseln

audience *20T* Publikum

Australian *18* Australier/in; australisch

author *77* Autor/in, Verfasser/in

authorities *pl 79* Behörden

automatic(ally) *72* automatisch

available *12* verfügbar, erhältlich; to **be ~ for sth** *82* für etw zur Verfügung stehen

average *12* Durchschnitt, Durchschnitts-

to **avoid** *55* vermeiden

awake, to **stay ~** *86* wach bleiben

award-winning *63* preisgekrönt

aware, to **be ~ about sth** *63* über etw Bescheid wissen

awful(ly) *46T* schrecklich, fürchterlich

B

baby food *57T* Babynahrung

back *32T* Rückseite, hinterer Teil

backache *35* Rückenschmerzen

backwards *83* rückwärts

ballpoint pen *27* Kugelschreiber

to **ban** *63* verbieten

bandage *35T* Verband; *38* Binde, Bandage

bath, relaxing ~ *86T* Entspannungsbad

beach *46T* Strand

to **bear** *22* tragen

to **beat** *42* schlagen

because of sth *65* wegen etw

beef *57T* Rind(fleisch)

beforehand *86T* vorher

to **begin:** to **~ with** *76* zunächst (einmal)

to **behave:** to **be badly ~ed** *56* sich schlecht benehmen, unartig sein

behaviour *76* Verhalten, Benehmen

to **believe** *37* glauben

below *9* unten(stehend)

benefit *49T* Nutzen, Vorteil

benign *74T* gutartig

besides *20T* außerdem

best, to **look one's ~** *20T* (möglichst) gut aussehen

to **bet** *49T* wetten

bike *30* Fahrrad

bill *22* Rechnung; to **settle a ~** *20T* eine Rechnung bezahlen

billion *66* Milliarde

to **binge** *67* sich vollstopfen; *76* sich vollsaufen

binge *67* Fressattacke; **~ drinking** *76* Komasaufen, Alkoholexzess

birth *18* Geburt; **date of ~** *18* Geburtsdatum

biscuit *57* Keks

black market *63* Schwarzmarkt

bladder *44* Harnblase; **~ wall** *44* Harnblasenwand

to **block sth from doing sth** *44* verhindern, daß etw etw tut

blocked *34T* verstopft

blood *6* Blut; **~ flow** *43* Blutstom, Durchblutung; **~ glucose control** *59* Blutzuckerregulation; **~ glucose level** *59* Blutzuckerspiegel; **high ~ pressure** *42* Bluthochdruck; **~ sample** *6* Blutprobe; **~ test** *16* Blutuntersuchung

blood-pressure cuff *38* Blutdruckmanschette

bloodstream *76* Blutkreislauf

blurred vision *52* verschwommenes Sehen

body weight *64T* Körpergewicht

boiled *68* gekocht

boiling *23T* kochend(heiß)

to **book** *12* reservieren, buchen

booking *9* Reservierung

booth *45* Kabine

boring *7* langweilig

both … and *12* sowohl … als auch

bra *73* BH

brachial artery *43* Oberarmarterie

brain *32* Gehirn, Hirn

to **brainstorm** *75* Ideen sammeln

bread roll *57* Brötchen

to **break sth** *30* sich etw brechen

breast *51T* Brust

to **breast-feed** *72T* stillen

breast-feeding *44* Stillen

to **breathe** *23T* atmen

broad *88* breit

broadband *45* Breitband

broken glass *39* Glasscherbe(n)

brush *51T* Bürste, Pinsel

bubble *63* Luftblase

build-up *42* Aufbau

bulb *43* Ballon

bulimia *64T* Bulimie

bulimic *64T* Bulimiker/in

burger van *63* Imbisswagen

to **burn a candle** *49T* eine Kerze verwenden, brennen lassen

business trip *20T* Geschäftsreise

busy, to **be ~** *15T* viel zu tun haben

C

cabbage *57T* Kohl

calculator *26* Taschenrechner

calendar *26* Kalender

to **call** *10* anrufen; **~** *37* rufen; **~ sb back** *17* jdn zurückrufen

call *17* (Telefon-)Anruf

called *10T* namens

caller *17* Anrufer/in

calm *7* ruhig

to **calm** *51* beruhigen

calorie *56* Kalorie

campaign *63* Kampagne

to **cancel** *21* absagen, stornieren

cancer *48* Krebs *(Krankheit);* **~-giving** *78* krebserregend

candidate *37* Kandidat/in

candle *49* Kerze; to **burn a ~** *49T* eine Kerze verwenden, brennen lassen

cannabinoid *79* Cannabinoid

canola *AE 57T* Raps

capsule *52* Kapsel

car crash *76* Autounfall

carbohydrates *pl 56* Kohlenhydrate

carbonated *63* mit Kohlensäure

card reader port *26* Kartenleseranschluss

cardiac *42* Herz-

cardiologist *37* Kardiologe/-in

cardiovascular *37* Herz-Kreislauf-, kardiovaskulär

care *7* Betreuung, Pflege; **~ assistant** *81* Pflegeassistent/in

care, to **take ~ of sb/sth** *22* sich um jdn/etw kümmern; *55* auf jdn/etw aufpassen, sich um jdn kümmern; **health ~** *7* Gesundheitswesen, medizinische

Versorgung; **Primary C~ Physician (PCP)** *AE* *7* Allgemeinarzt/-ärztin; **social ~** *55* Sozialfürsorge, Sozialdienste
to **care for sb** *81* jdn betreuen, sich um jdn kümmern, jdn pflegen
career *82T* Beruf, Laufbahn, Karriere; **~ ladder** *83* Karriereleiter
careers adviser *86* Berufsberater/in
careful(ly) *7* sorgfältig, genau
caring *12* sozial (eingestellt)
to **carry** *32T* befördern, transportieren; **~ out** *37* durchführen
cartridge *26* Kartusche, Patrone
case *17* Fall; **in ~** *17* für den Fall, dass; falls
cash, in ~ *22* (in) bar
to **catch sth** *48* sich mit etw anstecken
category *42* Klasse, Kategorie
catwalk *70* Laufsteg
to **cause** *33* verursachen
cause *37* Ursache; *44* Anlass
cell *51T* Zelle
cellar *20T* Keller
central nervous system *79* Zentrales Nervensystem
cereal *57* Getreide, Getreideflocken
certain *13* bestimmte/r/s
certificate *13* Urkunde, Abschluss(zeugnis), Zertifikat
certified *80* (staatlich) geprüft
cervix *51T* Gebärmutterhals
chain *35T* Kette
challenge *70* Herausforderung, Kampfansage, Wettstreit
challenging *12* fordernd, anspruchsvoll
to **change** *42* (sich) verändern, (sich) ändern
change *42* Änderung, Veränderung; *65* Gelegenheit, Chance; **~ of government** *63* Regierungswechsel
characteristic *80* Merkmal, Kennzeichen
charge *22* Gebühr(en), Kosten; *32* Ladung; **free of ~** *22* kostenlos; **prescription ~** *22* Rezeptgebühr
chart *57* Grafik; **flow ~** *75* Flussdiagramm
to **check** *8* überprüfen
check *AE* *22* Scheck
check-up *30* (Routine-)Untersuchung
cheerful *80* gut gelaunt, fröhlich
chef *63* Koch/Köchin, Küchenchef/in
chemist *79* Chemiker/in
chemistry *79* Chemie
chemotherapy *78* Chemotherapie
chest *23T* Brust; **~ infection** *61* Lungeninfekt
chicken *57* Huhn
childhood *66* Kindheit, Jugend; **~ obesity** *66* Fettleibigkeit bei Kindern und Jugendlichen
children's corner *49* Spielecke
Chinese *47* chinesisch
chips *BE* *63* Pommes frites
choice *8* Wahl, Auswahl
cholesterol *57T* Cholesterin; **~ level** *57T* Cholesterinspiegel
to **choose** *12* wählen, auswählen
to **circulate** *76* zirkulieren, fließen
circulation *64T* Durchblutung, (Blut-)Kreislauf
to **claim sth back** *22* etw zurückfordern
class *13* Unterricht, Kurs; **middle ~** *63* Mittelstand, zum Mittelstand gehörend
clause *68* Satzglied, Nebensatz
cleanliness *11* Sauberkeit
clear(ly) *17* deutlich
client *55* Klient/in, Kunde/Kundin
clinic *12* Klinik
clinical *13* klinisch; **~ assisting** *AE* *13* Behandlungsassistenz
close: ~ (to sth) *10T* nahe (bei etw); **~ by** *30* nahe gelegen; **~ to life** *45* lebensnah
clothes *pl* *23T* Kleider
clothing *43* Kleidung, Bekleidung; **upper ~** *73* Oberbekleidung
coach *59* Reisebus
coconut *57T* Kokosnuss; **~ oil** *57T* Kokosöl
cold *34* Erkältung
cold cut *57* Aufschnitt
coldness *48* Kälte
colleague *18* Kollege/-in
to **collect** *9* (ein)sammeln, kassieren; *52* abholen
colon *78* Dickdarm
coloured *27* bunt, farbig
to **come** *27* *(Waren:)* (es) geben, geliefert werden
comfort *70* Trost
comfortable *7* angenehm, behaglich; *11* bequem; to **feel ~** *48* sich wohlfühlen
command, good ~ *84* gute Beherrschung
common(ly) *13* üblich, gewöhnlich, verbreitet, häufig
communication *13* Kommunikation
community *45* Gemeinde; **~ college** *AE* *80* *weiterbildende und Berufsschule in den USA, die auch Erwachsenen offensteht*
to **compare** *41* vergleichen
compared with *37* verglichen mit
complaint, stomach ~s *pl* *52* Magenbeschwerden
to **complete** *8* vervollständigen; *18* *(Formular usw.)* ausfüllen
complete *9* vollständig; *75* abgeschlossen
to **complete sth** *13* etw abschließen, etw absolvieren; *83* etw *(Studium usw.)* abschließen
completely *51T* völlig, vollkommen
compound *79* (chemische) Verbindung
comprehensive school *84* Gesamtschule
to **concentrate** *20T* sich konzentrieren
concentration *56* Konzentration
to **concern** *75T* betreffen
concern *44* Besorgnis
condition *22* Leiden, Krankheit; *58* Zustand
to **conduct** *45* durchführen
confectionery foods *pl* *59* Süßwaren
confident *80* selbstbewusst
to **confirm** *17* bestätigen
to **connect** *45* verbinden
to **consider** *21* betrachten, in Betracht ziehen; **~ sth to be** *70* etw für etw halten
considered, to **be ~ sth** *63* als etw gelten
to **consist of sth** *11* aus etw bestehen
constant(ly) *71* ständig
constipation *70* Verstopfung
to **consult** *35* konsultieren; beraten
consultant *37* Facharzt/-ärztin
consultation, medical ~ *45* medizinische Beratung
to **consume** *57* verzehren; *76* konsumieren
consumption *68* Verzehr, Konsum, Verbrauch
contagious *59* ansteckend
to **contain** *56* enthalten
to **continue: ~ sth** *75T* mit etw weitermachen; **~ to do sth** *43* etw weiter(hin) tun
to **contract** *42* sich zusammenziehen
control, to **be in ~ of sth** *67* etw unter Kontrolle haben
to **cope with sth** *78* mit etw fertigwerden, mit etw klarkommen
copier *26* Kopierer, Kopiergerät
to **copy** *19* abschreiben; *66T* nachahmen
copy *26* Kopie; *75T* Exemplar
corner *10T* Ecke; **children's ~** *49* Spielecke

coronary heart disease 37 koronare Herzerkrankung
correlation 78 Wechselbeziehung
correspondence 13 Schriftverkehr, Korrespondenz
corridor 25T Flur
cortex, prefrontal ~ 76 präfrontale Cortex
cotton 38 Baumwolle
cottonwool 41T Watte
cough 23T Husten
to **cough** 34T husten
council 81 Rat
to **counsel** 66 beraten
counselling 65 Beratung, Therapie
course 12 Kurs, Studiengang; **vocational ~** 80 Berufsbildungskurs
coursework 13 Studieninhalt, Studienumfang
courtesy 17 Höflichkeit
to **cover** 11 bedecken, verhüllen; 13 (ab)decken, *(Thema)* behandeln
coverage, insurance ~ 22 Versicherungsschutz
covered in sth 60 *hier:* mit etw überzogen
covering, head ~ 11 Kopfbedeckung
cranberry 44 Großfrüchtige Moosbeere, Kranbeere
crash: ~ diet 70 Radikalkur, Radikaldiät; **car ~** 76 Autounfall
crazy 61 verrückt
cream 57 Sahne
to **create** 45 schaffen
credit card 22 Kreditkarte
crew 70 Team
crisis, hypertensive ~ 42 hypertensive Krise
crisps *BE* 63 Chips
crowd 87 Masse, (Menschen-)Menge
crutches *pl* 30 Krücken
to **cry** 23T weinen, heulen
cuff 43 Manschette; **blood-pressure ~** 38 Blutdruckmanschette
cultivated 11 kultiviert
cultural 47 kulturell
culture 7 Kultur
current 22 aktuell
currently 82 derzeit, zurzeit, momentan
curriculum vitae (CV) 82 Lebenslauf
curvy 70 kurvig
customer 18 Kunde/-in; **~ reference number** 27 Kundennummer
cut 30 Schnitt, Schnittwunde, Schnittverletzung; **cold ~** 57 Aufschnitt
to **cut back** 70 kürzen, zurückschrauben
cycle 72T Zyklus
cyst 73 Zyste

D

daily 7 täglich
dairy products 57 Molkereiprodukte, Milchprodukte
damage 61 Schaden, Schäden
to **damage** 76 beschädigen
date, up to ~ 7 auf dem neuesten Stand, aktuell; **out of ~** 83 veraltet; **~ of birth** 18 Geburtsdatum
deadly 79 tödlich
deaf 30 taub
to **deal: ~ with sb** 17 mit jdm umgehen, gegenüber jdm auftreten; **~ with sth** 17 mit etw umgehen, etw erledigen, etw bearbeiten; 37 mit etw zu tun haben; 64T mit etw fertigwerden, etw bewältigen; 65 sich mit etw befassen
death 47 Tod; 60 Todesfall
decision 76 Entscheidung; to **make a ~** 76 eine Entscheidung fällen; **~-making** 81 Entscheidungsfindung
to **decrease** 60 abnehmen, sinken; **~ sth** 44 etw senken, etw reduzieren
to **define** 75 definieren
to **deflate sth** 43 Luft aus etw lassen
degree 13 Abschluss; **associate ~** *AE* 13 *US-Abschluss, der nach zwei Jahren verliehen wird*
to **delay** 76 verzögern
delivery 13 Umsetzung, Anwendung; **~ note** 25T Lieferschein
dental 47 Zahn-
department store 82 Kaufhaus
to **depend on sth** 11 von etw abhängen
dependence 75T Abhängigkeit
depressed 64T deprimiert
depression 37 Depression
to **describe** 7 beschreiben
to **design** 37 gestalten, entwerfen
designed, to **be ~ to do sth** 81 dafür gedacht sein, etw zu tun
desirable 81 erwünscht
desk, front ~ 7 Rezeption, Anmeldung
despite 63 trotz
detail, in ~ 51T im Einzelnen, detailliert
details *pl* 8 Angaben, Daten
to **develop** 37 entwickeln
development 37 Entwicklung
device 45 Gerät
diabetes 37 Diabetes
diabetic 60 Diabetes-
to **diagnose** 9 diagnostizieren; **~ sb with sth** 59 etw *(Krankheit)* bei jdm feststellen
diagnosis, to **make a ~** 33 eine Diagnose stellen
diagram 32 Grafik
diarrhoea 34T Durchfall
diastolic 42 diastolisch
to **die (from sth)** 37 (an etw) sterben
diet 56 Ernährung, Kost; 70 Diät; **crash ~** 70 Radikalkur, Radikaldiät
dietary supplement 44 Nahrungsergänzungsmittel
dieting 65 eine Diät machen, Diät(en)
difference 13 Unterschied; to **make a ~** 42 etwas/viel ausmachen
difficulty 47 Schwierigkeit
dignity 55T Würde
diploma 12 Diplom
to **direct** 44 anweisen; **~ sb to sth** 21 jdn auf etw verweisen, jdn umleiten
directions *pl* 10 Wegbeschreibung; to **ask for ~** 25 nach dem Weg fragen; to **give ~** 10 den Weg beschreiben
director 37 Direktor/in
disabled 47 behindert
disadvantage 45 Nachteil
to **disagree** 34 nicht zustimmen
disaster 70 Katastrophe
discomfort 51T Unbehagen, leichter Schmerz
disconnected, to **get ~** 17 *(Telefonverbindung:)* unterbrochen werden
disease 37 Erkrankung, Krankheit; **coronary heart ~** 37 koronare Herzerkrankung; **sexually transmitted ~ (STD)** 76 sexuell übertragbare Krankheit
to **disinfect** 35T desinfizieren
disinfectant 38 Desinfektionsmittel
disorder 64 Störung; **alcohol-use ~** 75T alkoholbezogene Störung; **eating ~** 64 Essstörung
dissimilar (to sth) 79 (von etw) verschieden
to **dissolve** 52 auflösen; to **allow to ~** 52 zergehen lassen
distant 48 distanziert
distress 51 Kummer, Sorge
divided by 64 geteilt durch
dizzy 37 schwindlig
doctor, duty ~ 21 diensthabende/r Arzt/Ärztin; **family ~** 64T Hausarzt/Hausärztin
doctor's office *AE* 7 (Arzt-)Praxis
document 26 Dokument
documentation 13 Unterlagen, Dokumentation
dosage 52 Dosierung

dosing instructions *pl* *44* Dosierungsanleitung
dosis *44* Dosis, Gabe
to **double** *66* sich verdoppeln
to **double-check** *43* nochmals kontrollieren
to **down** *76* *(Getränk)* hinunterkippen
to **draw** *10* zeichnen
drawstring *11* Tunnelzug
to **dress** *39* *(Wunde)* verbinden
dress *11* Kleidung, Kleid; **~ code** *11* Bekleidungsvorschrift(en); **~ size** *70* Kleidergröße
dressed, to **get ~** *74T* sich anziehen
dressing *35* Verband
dried *44* getrocknet, Trocken-
driving licence *84* Führerschein
drop *63* Rückgang
drowsiness *52* Schläfrigkeit
drug *29T* Arzneimittel; *76* Droge; **~ user** *79* Drogenabhängige/r
drunk *76* betrunken
due to *14* aufgrund von
duty *6* Aufgabe; **~ doctor** *21* diensthabende/r Arzt/Ärztin

E

earache *35* Ohrenschmerzen
earring *11* Ohrring
ear wax *30* Ohrenschmalz
eating: ~ disorder *64* Essstörung; **~ habits** *pl* *63* Essgewohnheiten
economic *60* wirtschaftlich, ökonomisch
education *13* Schulbildung, Bildung
effect *63* Auswirkung(en), Folge; to **take ~** *39T* wirken; **knock-on ~** *78* Folgewirkung; **side ~** *52* Nebenwirkung
effective *44* wirksam
either … or *12* entweder … oder
elastic *38* elastisch
elderly people *81* ältere Menschen, Senioren
electrical *32* elektrisch
electrocardiograph (ECG) *32* Elektrokardiogramm (EKG)
electroencephalograph (EEG) *32* Elektroenzephalogramm (EEG)
electronic *9* elektronisch; **~ appointment book** *26* elektronischer Terminkalender
to **embark on sth** *63* etw in Angriff nehmen
emergency *13* Notfall
emotion *65* Gefühl(säußerung), Emotion
emotional *65* emotional, gefühlsmäßig
to **employ sb** *13* jdn einstellen, jdn beschäftigen
employee *86* Angestellte/r
employer *83* Arbeitgeber/in; **~ agency** *86* Arbeitsvermittlung
empty *52* leer
to **enable** *21* ermöglichen, befähigen
enc(losures *pl***)** *82* *(Brief:)* Anlagen
enclosed *82* *(Brief:)* beigefügt
to **encourage** *65* fördern; *65* ermutigen, ermuntern
end, to **see an ~ to sth** *63* mit etw ein Ende machen
endocannabinoid *79* Endocannabinoid
to **endure sth** *78* etw ertragen, etw erleiden
to **enjoy** *55T* genießen, gern tun; **~ doing sth** *7* etw gern tun
to **enter a room** *87* ein Zimmer betreten
enthusiasm *64T* Begeisterung
enthusiastic about sth *81* von etw begeistert
to **entitle sb to sth** *14* jdm einen Anspruch auf etw verleihen
environment *12* Umfeld
environmental *59* Umwelt-
equal, to **be ~ to sth** *60* entsprechen
equally *59* gleich, gleichermaßen
equipment *6* Ausstattung, Geräte; **office ~** *26* Büroausstattung, Bürobedarf; **piece of ~** *39* Gerät, Utensil
equipped, to **be ~ with sth** *13* mit etw ausgestattet sein, über etw verfügen
equivalent *84* Entsprechung
especially *17* besonders
essential *55T* wesentlich, notwendig
to **estimate** *60* schätzen
ethics *13* Ethik
etiquette *17* Anstandsregel, Etikette
European Economic Area *14* Europäischer Wirtschaftsraum
even *18* sogar; **~ though** *70* obwohl
everyday *68* Alltags-, alltäglich
evidence *81* Nachweis
evident *78* deutlich, offensichtlich
exam *12* Prüfung; *35* Untersuchung; to **take an ~** *47* eine Prüfung machen
examination *12* Prüfung; *35* Untersuchung; **pelvic ~** *46T* gynäkologische Untersuchung; **~ gloves** *pl* *38* Untersuchungshandschuhe; **~ table** *73* Untersuchungsliege
to **examine** *35* untersuchen
excellent *9* ausgezeichnet, hervorragend
excess *63* überschüssig
excited *70* aufgeregt, freudig erregt
exciting *7* spannend, aufregend
exercise *42* Bewegung, (Ausgleichs-) Sport; to **do ~** *59* sich bewegen, Sport treiben
to **expect (sb to do sth)** *49T* erwarten (dass jd etw tut)
expectation *65* Erwartung; to **meet ~s** *67* Erwartungen erfüllen
experience *13* Erfahrung; *45* Erlebnis
to **experience sth** *66* etw erleben
experienced *81* erfahren
experiment *45* Versuch, Experiment
to **experiment** *76* experimentieren
explanation *47* Erklärung, Erläuterung
to **express** *47* ausdrücken
expression *8* Ausdruck
extended *21* ausgeweitet, erweitert
extension *20T* *(Telefon:)* Durchwahl
extra *21* zusätzlich
to **extract** *39* herausziehen
extraordinary *63* außerordentlich
extreme(ly) *42* extrem

F

face-to-face *45* direkt, persönlich
facial hair *64T* Gesichtsbehaarung
facility *65* Einrichtung
fact, in ~ *27* in der Tat, tatsächlich, eigentlich
factor *37* Faktor
to **fade** *43* schwächer werden, verklingen
to **fail** *63* scheitern
failure *65* Scheitern, Versagen
to **fall behind** *76* zurückfallen
family doctor *64T* Hausarzt/Hausärztin
far, as ~ as *33* soweit
fat *57* Fett; **saturated ~s** *pl* *57T* gesättigte Fettsäure
fatal *76* tödlich
favour, to **do sb a ~** *20T* jdm einen Gefallen tun
fear (of sth) *47* Furcht, Angst (vor etw)
to **feature** *71* *(in einer Zeitschrift)* bringen
fee *9* Honorar, Gebühr
to **feed sb** *63* jdm zu essen geben
feeling *13* Gefühl, Ansicht, Meinung
fever *23T* Fieber
fibre *57T* Ballaststoff; **high-~** *57T* ballaststoffreich
field, in the ~ *13* in der Praxis
to **fight sb** *67* jdn bekämpfen, gegen jnd kämpfen
final *75T* letzte/r/s
finally *29T* zuletzt, als letztes, schließlich
financial injection *63* finanzielle Unterstützung, Finanzspritze

to **find: you may ~** *7* es kann sein, es kann vorkommen; **~ out** *22* herausfinden
fingernails *pl*, **trimmed ~** *11* kurze Fingernägel
first: ~ aid *13* Erste Hilfe; **~ name** *18* Vorname; **at ~** *74T* zunächst
to **fit** *43* passen, sitzen; **~ sb in** *14* *(Termin:)* jdn einschieben, jdn dazwischenschieben
fizzy drink *63* kohlensäurehaltige Limonade
flat *70* flach
flexible *87* flexibel
flight *20T* Flug
flooded *20T* überschwemmt
floor plan *25* Grundriss
flow: blood ~ *43* Blutstom, Durchblutung; **~ chart** *75* Flussdiagramm
flu *34* Grippe; **~ jab** *59* Grippe(schutz) impfung
fluids *pl* *33* Flüssigkeit
foetus *57T* Fötus
folic acid *57T* Folsäure
follow-up *75T* Folge-
following *7* folgende/r/s
food: ~ poisoning *34* Lebensmittelvergiftung; **F~ and Drug Administration (FDA)** *44 US-Behörde für Arznei- und Lebensmittelzulassung;* **baby ~** *57T* Babynahrung; **confectionery ~s** *pl* *59* Süßwaren; to **keep ~ down** *35* Essen bei sich behalten
foot spa *49* Fußbad
footwear *11* Schuhe, Schuhwerk
force *72* Kraft
foreign *16* ausländisch, aus dem Ausland; **~ language skills** *pl* *83* Fremdsprachenkenntnisse
formal *18* formal, förmlich, formell
foundation *37* Stiftung; *65* Fundament
free: to **be ~** *23T* Zeit haben; **~ of charge** *22* kostenlos
frequent *42* häufig
fresh *58* frisch
fried egg *68* Spiegelei
friend, to **make ~s** *86* Freunde finden
friendliness *11* Freundlichkeit
front *32T* Vorderseite, vorderer Teil; **~ desk** *7* Rezeption, Anmeldung; **~ line** *12* an vorderster Front
frustrated *55T* frustriert
full: in ~ *22* vollständig, in voller Höhe; **~ fat milk** *58* Vollmilch
full-time *12* Vollzeit-
fully *49* vollständig
function *32* Funktion
funding *63* Finanzierung
further *17* weitere/r/s
fuss, to **make a ~** *72T* sich anstellen, Theater machen
future *88* zukünftig, für die Zukunft

G
to **gain a pass** *12* eine Prüfung bestehen
gate *63* Tor
gauge *43* Messgerät, *hier:* Manometer
gauze *38* Gaze, Verbandmull
gel, acoustic ~ *74* Ultraschallgel
general *7* allgemein; **in ~** *18* im Allgmeinen; **~ practice** *12* Allgemeinarztpraxis; **~ practice nurse** *BE* *80* *brit. Arzthelfer/in, die ausschließlich Behandlungsaufgaben erledigt;* **G~ Practitioner (GP)** *BE* *7* Allgemeinarzt/-ärztin
generally *65* im Allgemeinen
genetic *59* genetisch, erblich
gentle *51T* behutsam; *73* sanft
germ *46T* Keim, Bakterie
to **get: ~ in the way of sth** *43* einer Sache im Wege sein; **~ up** *24* aufstehen
glad *41T* froh
gland *33* Drüse
glass, broken ~ *39* Glasscherbe(n)
global *60* weltweit, global
glossy magazine *64T* Hochglanzmagazin
gloves *pl*, **examination ~** *38* Untersuchungshandschuhe
glucose, blood ~ control *59* Blutzuckerregulation; **blood ~ level** *59* Blutzuckerspiegel
goal *75T* Ziel
gold medal *59* Goldmedaille
government *63* Regierung; **change of ~** *63* Regierungswechsel
graduate *79* Absolvent/in
grain *58* Korn, Getreide
grateful *20T* dankbar
greasy *11* fettig
to **greet** *9* begrüßen
grey matter *76* die grauen Zellen
to **grow** *70* wachsen, werden
growing *63* wachsend, zunehmend, steigend
growth *64T* Wachstum, Wuchs
guidelines *pl* *63* Richtlinien
guilt *67* Schuld
guilty *68* schuldig
gullet *32* Speiseröhre
gynaecologist *30* Gynäkologe/-in

H
habits *pl*, **eating ~** *63* Essgewohnheiten
hair loss *64T* Haarausfall
hallucination *79* Wahnvorstellung(en), Halluzination(en)
hand, on the other ~ *79* andererseits
to **hand sth out** *75T* etw austeilen
hand-written *83* handgeschrieben
to **handle** *81* erledigen
handout *75T* Arbeitsblatt, Informationsblatt
hands-on *45* praktisch, direkt
to **hang out with sb** *66T* mit jdm abhängen
happen *23T* passieren, geschehen
happy, to **be ~ to do sth** *17* etw gern tun
to **harm** *57T* schädigen, schaden
harmful *57T* schädlich
hat *11* Haube, Mütze, Kappe
to **hate** *48* hassen, überhaupt nicht mögen
head covering *11* Kopfbedeckung
headache *34T* Kopfschmerzen
heading *47* Überschrift
to **head: ~ing south** *10T* in Richtung Süden
to **heal** *35T* heilen, verheilen
health: ~ care *7* Gesundheitswesen, medizinische Versorgung; **~ centre** *7* Gesundheitszentrum; **~ insurance** *7* Krankenversicherung; **National H~ Service (NHS)** *21* Staatlicher Gesundheitsdienst; **World H~ Organization (WHO)** *70* Weltgesundheitsorganisation
healthy *56* gesund
hearing aid *47* Hörgerät
heart *32* Herz; **~ attack** *37* Herzinfarkt; **~ disease** *37* Herzerkrankung; **~ rate** *37* Puls, Herzfrequenz
heartbeat *39* Herzschlag
heavy *75T* schwer
height *64* Körpergröße
helpful *73* hilfreich, nützlich
helpfulness *11* Hilfsbereitschaft
helpless *48* hilflos
helplessness *55T* Hilflosigkeit
hepatitis *41T* Hepatitis
herbal *44* Kräuter-, Pflanzen-
high *33* *hier:* erhöht; *67* Hochgefühl; to **be ~ in sth** *57T* einen hohen Anteil von etw haben; **~ blood pressure** *42* Bluthochdruck
high-definition *45* hochauflösend
high-fibre *57T* ballaststoffreich
high-profile *63* öffentlichkeitswirksam

high-risk patient *75T* Risikopatient
highly qualified *80* hochqualifiziert
history, medical ~ *18* Krankengeschichte
hives *pl* *44* Nesselsucht
hold, to **put sb on ~** *17* *(Telefon:)* jdn in die Warteschleife stellen
to **hold out** *35T* hinhalten
holiday, public ~ *20T* (gesetzlicher) Feiertag
home visit *23T* Hausbesuch
honest *55* ehrlich, aufrichtig
honesty *55T* Ehrlichkeit, Aufrichtigkeit
honey *58* Honig
hopelessness *67* Hoffnungslosigkeit
horrible *64T* schrecklich, furchtbar
hours *pl* *21* Öffnungszeiten, Sprechzeiten; **out of ~** *21* außerhalb der Geschäfts-/Sprechzeiten
huge *79* riesengroß, riesig
human *51* human, menschlich
humiliation *65* Demütigung
to **hurt** *23T* wehtun; *76* verletzen; **~ oneself** *23T* sich wehtun, sich verletzen
hygiene, personal ~ *11* Körperpflege
hypertension *42* Hypertonie
hypertensive crisis *42* hypertensive Krise
hypodermic (syringe) *38* Injektionsspritze

I

ID card *25T* Personalausweis
to **identify** *17* identifizieren, genau bestimmen
if: ~ so *29T* falls ja; **as ~** *45* als ob
to **ignore** *65* ignorieren
ill-tempered *55T* griesgrämig, verärgert
illegal(ly) *63* illegal
illness *14* Krankheit
image *17* Bild (in der Öffentlichkeit), Image; *45* Bild
to **imagine** *79* sich (etw) vorstellen
immediate(ly) *42* unverzüglich, sofortig
immune system *70* Immunsystem
immunization *41* Schutzimpfung, Immunisierung
to **impose sth** *79* etw durchsetzen
impression *12* Eindruck
to **improve** *58* (sich) bessern, verbessern
improvement *49* Verbesserung
in, one ~ five *66T* eine/r/s von fünf
inappropriate *76* unangemessen
to **include** *13* einschließen, beinhalten
including *13* einschließlich
incontinence *44* Inkontinenz
to **inconvenience sb** *14* jdm Unannehmlichkeiten bereiten
incorrect *60* falsch
increase *78* Zunahme
to **increase** *57T* erhöhen; *78* zunehmen, steigen
increased *76* erhöht
increasing *42* zunehmend
incredible *66T* unglaublich
to **indicate** *83* angeben
individual *8* Individuum
infection *24* Infektion; *47* Ansteckung
infectious *60* ansteckend
infirmary *45* Krankenhaus
inflamed *33* entzündet
to **inflate** *43* aufpumpen
ingredient *79* Bestandteil
initials *pl* *79* Initialen
to **inject** *39* injizieren
injection *9* Injektion, Spritze; **financial ~** *63* finanzielle Unterstützung, Finanzspritze
to **injure** *76* verletzen
injury *11* Verletzung
inquiry *81* Anfrage
insecure *70* unsicher, verunsichert
instance, for ~ *76* zum Beispiel
institution *11* Einrichtung, Institution
instruction *13* Unterricht; *52* Anleitung; *73* Aufforderung; **dosing ~s** *pl* *44* Dosierungsanleitung
insulin *59* Insulin
insurance *7* Versicherung; **health ~** *7* Krankenversicherung; **~ coverage** *22* Versicherungsschutz
intake *56* Zufuhr
to **interact with sth** *75T* eine Wechselwirkung mit etw haben
interactive *79* kommunikativ
intermediate *12* mittel, Zwischen-; **~ French** *84* Französisch auf fortgeschrittenem Anfängerniveau
intern *87* Praktikant/in
internal *51T* innere/r/s
internship *13* Praktikum
interpersonal skills *pl* *81* soziale Kompetenz
interview, job ~ *47* Vorstellungsgespräch
interviewee *86* Befragte/r, Bewerber(in)
interviewer *86* jd, der ein Vorstellungsgespräch führt
to **introduce** *63* einführen
introduction *63* Einführung
invasive *49* invasiv
to **invite** *72* einladen
invoice *7* Rechnung
to **involve** *48* mit sich bringen, einschließen
involved, to **be ~ in sth** *12* an etw beteiligt sein, mit etw zu tun haben
irregular *64T* unregelmäßig
issue *75* Problem
itching *44* Juckreiz
item *11* Gegenstand; *22* Artikel

J

jab, flu ~ *59* Grippe(schutz)impfung
jacket *41* Jacke
jar *58* Glas
jealous (of sth) *70* eifersüchtig (auf etw), neidisch (auf etw)
jewellery *86T* Schmuck
jigsaw puzzle *45* Puzzle
job: ~ advertisment *81* Stellenanzeige, -ausschreibung; **~ interview** *47* Vorstellungsgespräch
to **join: ~ sb** *66T* zu jdm gehen, sich zu jdm gesellen; **~ sb/sth** *87* bei jdm/etw mitmachen, sich jdm/einer Sache anschließen
joint *35* Gelenk
journal *67* Zeitschrift
joy (of sth) *70* Freude (über etw)
juice *57* Saft

K

to **keep: ~ doing sth** *34T* etw die ganze Zeit tun; **~ up** *76* Schritt halten; **~ food down** *35* Essen bei sich behalten; **~ records** *6* Akten halten, Unterlagen führen
key *13* wichtigste/r/s, ausschlaggebend
to **key in** *19* eintippen, *(Daten)* eingeben
keyboard *26* Tastatur
to **kick in** *70* einsetzen
kid *46T* Kind
kidney *79* Niere; **~ stones** *pl* *44*
killer *58* Todesursache
kind *29T* Art
knock-on effect *78* Folgewirkung
knowledge *12* Wissen, Kenntnisse

L

lab(oratory) *7* Labor
to **label** *25* etikettieren, bezeichnen
label *26* Etikett
lack *78* Mangel
ladder, career ~ *83* Karriereleiter
to **launch sth** *87* etw starten
law *13* Recht, Gesetz(e)
laxative *64T* Abführmittel
lazy *55T* faul

to **lead** *59* führen
lead, in the ~ *79* ganz vorn
leading *78* Haupt-, führend
leaflet *37* Broschüre, Merkblatt
to **leap** *78* sprunghaft ansteigen
to **leave school** *31* von der Schule abgehen
legal age, minimum ~ *76* gesetzliches Mindestalter
length *12* Länge
lesson *45* Lehre, Lektion
letter of application *82* Bewerbungsschreiben
lettuce leaves *pl* *70* Salatblätter
leukaemia *78* Blutkrebs, Leukämie
level *80* Stufe, Ebene; **blood glucose ~** *59* Blutzuckerspiegel; **cholesterol ~** *57T* Cholesterinspiegel; **mineral ~s** *70* Mineralstoffgehalt; **stock ~s** *84* Lagerbestände
licence, driving ~ *84* Führerschein
licensed practical nurse *AE* *80* staatlich geprüfte/r Krankenpflegehelfer/in
to **lie: ~ around** *50* herumliegen; **~ down** *51T* sich hinlegen
life: to **take your ~** *67* sich umbringen; **~ history** *83* Lebensgeschichte
life-size *45* lebensgroß
life-threatening *21* lebensbedrohlich
lifestyle *42* Lebensweise
likely *42* wahrscheinlich
to **limit** *57T* begrenzen, beschränken
limit *75T* Höchstgrenze, Grenzwert
lip *32T* Lippe
to **list** *67* (in einer Liste) aufführen
listener *80* Zuhörer/in
to **live up to sth** *65* einer Sache gerecht werden, etw erfüllen
liver *75T* Leber
local *21* ortsansässig, örtlich; to **give a ~ anaesthetic** *39* örtlich betäuben
to **locate** *43* ausfindig machen
lonely *55T* einsam
long-lasting *79* dauerhaft
long-term *42* langfristig
longer-term *77* längerfristig
look, to **have/take a ~** *14* nachsehen, sich etw ansehen
to **look: ~ after sb** *6* sich um jdn kümmern; **~ forward to sth** *82* sich auf etw freuen; **~ one's best** *20T* (möglichst) gut aussehen
loose *11* *(Kleidung:)* weit
to **lose weight** *59* abnehmen
loss *44* Verlust; **weight ~** *64T* Gewichtsverlust, -abnahme
lower *42* untere/r/s
lump *72T* Knoten
lungs *pl* *32T* Lunge

M

machine *73* Gerät
madness *70* Irrsinn
magazine *9* Zeitschrift
main *10T* Haupt-
mainly *37* hauptsächlich
to **maintain** *11* halten, behalten, beibehalten
major *32T* Haupt-
to **make: ~ (it)** *15* (es) schaffen; **~ sb do sth** *7* jdn dazu bringen, etw zu tun; **~ sth up** *51* sich etw ausdenken, etw erfinden; **~ sure** *7* dafür sorgen; **~ a fuss** *72T* sich anstellen, Theater machen; **~ friends** *86* Freunde finden; **~ use of sth** *82T* etw nutzen, sich etw zunutze machen
malignant *74T* bösartig
malnutrition *64T* Unterernährung
mammogram *72T* Mammographie
to **manage** *26* verwalten, organisieren; *79* (es) schaffen
manager *55T* Geschäftsführer/in
map *10* Karte, Plan
maple syrup *57* Ahornsirup
marijuana *79* Marihuana
marital status *83* Familienstand
to **mark** *10* markieren, kennzeichnen; **~ sth** *74T* auf etw Flecken hinterlassen
to **marry** *82* heiraten
to **massage** *49* massieren
massage *49T* Massage
to **match** *6* zuordnen; **~ sth to sth** *86T* etw an etw anpassen
matter, grey ~ *76* die grauen Zellen
mature *12* *hier:* älter/e
meal *33* Mahlzeit
to **mean** *14* bedeuten, heißen
measles *pl* *34* Masern
to **measure** *32* messen
meat *57* Fleisch
medal, gold ~ *59* Goldmedaille
medical *7* medizinisch, ärztlich; **~ administrator** *12* Arzthelfer/in (für Verwaltungsaufgaben); **~ assistant** *6* Medizinische Fachangestellte/r; **~ attention** *65* ärztliche Behandlung, ärztliche Hilfe; **~ card** *22* Gesundheitskarte; **condition** *22* Leiden, Krankheit; **~ consultation** *45* medizinische Beratung; **~ history** *18* Krankengeschichte; **~ office** *AE* *13* (Arzt-)Praxis; **~ receptionist** *9* Sprechstundenhilfe; **~ secretary** *12* Arzthelfer/in (für Organisationsaufgaben); **~ supplies** *pl* *9* Sanitätsartikel
medication *29T* Medikamente
medicine *24* Arzneimittel; *49T* Medizin
to **meet expectations** *67* Erwartungen erfüllen
meeting *23T* Sitzung, Besprechung, Treffen
member *12* Mitglied
membership *81* Mitgliedschaft; **~ organization** *81* Fachverband, Berufsverband
menopause *37* Wechseljahre, Menopause
menstruation *72* Menstruation
mental *47* geistig
to **mention sth** *87* etw erwähnen
mercury *42* Quecksilber
message *17* Mitteilung, Nachricht; to **take a ~** *17* *(Telefon:)* etw ausrichten
middle class *63* Mittelstand, zum Mittelstand gehörend
middle-aged *37* mittleren Alters
midwifery *81* Geburtshilfe
migraine *30* Kopfschmerzen, Migräne
mild *37* leicht
mile *31* Meile
milk: full fat ~ *58* Vollmilch; **skimmed ~** *58* entrahmte Milch; **whole ~** *68* Vollmilch
mind *67* Verstand, Geist, Kopf
to **mind** *82T* etw dagegen haben; **Never ~.** *34T* Macht nichts.
mineral levels *pl* *70* Mineralstoffgehalt
to **minimize** *11* auf ein Mindestmaß reduzieren/beschränken
minimum *76* Mindest-, mindestens; **~ legal age** *76* gesetzliches Mindestalter
minor *7* klein; *44* gering, geringfügig
minority *52* Minderzahl
miserable *70* elend
to **miss: ~ sth** *44* etw versäumen; *65* etw verpassen; **~ out on sth** *83* sich etw entgehen lassen
missing *19* fehlend
mixed up *70* durcheinander, vertauscht
mobile phone *83* Mobiltelefon
moderation, in ~ *78* in Maßen, maßvoll
to **monitor** *42* überwachen
mood swing *65* Stimmungsschwankung
motivate *83* motivieren
motivation *67* Motivation
to **move** *31* umziehen; *45* verlegen; **~ house** *7* umziehen
muscle *42* Muskel

a must 83 ein Muss

N

name, by ~ 17 namentlich; **first ~** 18 Vorname
nasal passage 32 Nasengang
national 61 Staatsbürger/in; **N~ Health Service (NHS)** 21 Staatlicher Gesundheitsdienst
nationality 83 Staatsangehörigkeit
nationally set 12 landesweit einheitlich
native speaker 84 Muttersprachler/in
nausea 52 Übelkeit
necessarily, not ~ 42 nicht unbedingt
neck 33 Hals, Nacken
need 22 Bedürfnis
needle 38 Nadel
needle-holder 38 Nadelhalter
needle-thread combination 38 Nadel-Faden-Kombination
nerve 61 Nerv; **olfactory ~** 32 Geruchsnerv
nerve-racking 88 nervenaufreibend
nervous 29T aufgeregt, nervös
nervousness 87 Aufregung, Nervosität
nervous system, central ~ 79 Zentrales Nervensystem
network 45 Netzwerk
news *pl* 47 Neuigkeiten, Nachrichten
non-nutritional 63 nährwertlos
nonprescription 44 nicht rezeptpflichtig, rezeptfrei
normally 18 normalerweise
north 10T Norden
northern 10T nördlich, Nord-
note 7 Notiz; to **take ~s** 7 (sich) Notizen machen
to **note** 12 notieren, aufschreiben
to **notice** 34T bemerken
nowadays 49 heutzutage
nurse 9 Krankenschwester/-pfleger; **general practice ~** *BE* 80 *brit. Arzthelfer/in, die ausschließlich Behandlungsaufgaben erledigt;* **licensed practical ~** *AE* 80 staatlich geprüfte/r Krankenpflegehelfer/in; **registered ~** 80 examinierte/r Krankenschwester/-pfleger; **staff ~** 81 examinierte/r Krankenschwester/-pfleger
nursing 81 Krankenpflege; **~ assistant** 80 Pflegehelfer/in; **~ home** 81 Pflegeheim
nutrition 56 Ernährung
nutritional 65 Ernährungs-; **non-~** 63 nährwertlos

O

oak 81 Eiche
obese 56 fettleibig
obesity 37 Fettleibigkeit
objective 48 objektiv
to **obsess about sth** 66 sich andauernd/zwanghaft mit etw beschäftigen
obviously 78 natürlich, selbstverständlich
occasional(ly) 21 gelegentlich
to **occur** 44 *(Ereignis:)* auftreten
the odd one out 8 *etwas, was nicht dazugehört*
odour 44 (übler) Geruch
oesophagus 32 Oesophagus
oestrogen 37 Östrogen
off, to **take a day ~ work** 46T sich einen Tag frei nehmen; to **take time ~** 55T sich freinehmen, sich Zeit nehmen
to **offer** 17 anbieten
offer, special ~ 27 Sonderangebot
office, doctor's ~ *AE* 7 (Arzt-)Praxis; **medical ~** *AE* 13 (Arzt-)Praxis; **~ equipment** 26 Büroausstattung, Bürobedarf
oil 57 Öl; **coconut ~** 57T Kokosöl; **palm ~** 57T Palmöl; **vegetable ~** 57T Pflanzenöl
old-fashioned 83 altmodisch
olfactory nerve 32 Geruchsnerv
olive 57T Olive
on-site 13 vor Ort
once 52 einmal
ongoing 45 laufend, andauernd
onion 57 Zwiebel
open, in the ~ 65 offen
open-toed 11 *(Schuhe:)* vorne offen
operation 7 Operation
opinion 12 Meinung, Ansicht
opposite 10 gegenüber; 60 Gegenteil
order 27 Bestellung, Auftrag; 43 Reihenfolge; **in ~ to** 7 um … zu
to **order** 7 bestellen, in Auftrag geben
organ 32T Organ
to **organise** 7 organisieren
organization 12 Organisation, Unternehmen, Verband; **membership ~** 81 Fachverband, Berufsverband
organizational 81 organisatorisch, Organisations-
otherwise 52 anders
otoscope 38 Ohrenspiegel, Otoskop
out: ~ of date 83 veraltet; **~ of hours** 21 außerhalb der Geschäfts-/Sprechzeiten
to **outline** 52 (kurz) darstellen, umreißen
outside 21 außerhalb; 74T Außenseite
overdose 79 Überdosis
to **overeat** 64T zu viel essen, sich überfressen
overeating 64T übermäßiges Essen
overweight 37 übergewichtig
overworked 37 überarbeitet
ovulation 72 Eisprung, Ovulation

P

pack 27 Packung
paediatrician 30 Kinderarzt/-ärztin
pain 16 Schmerz(en); to **be in ~** 16 Schmerzen haben
painful 23T schmerzhaft
painless 49T schmerzlos
pair, in ~s 23 paarweise
to **pair sth with sth** 11 etw mit etw kombinieren
palate 32 Gaumen
palm oil 57T Palmöl
to **panic** 74T in Panik geraten
pants *pl AE* 11 (lange) Hose
paperless 81 papierfrei
paperwork 7 Büroarbeit, Schreibarbeit(en); to **do ~** 7 Papierkram erledigen
papilloma virus 51 Papillomvirus
paragraph 47 *(Text:)* Absatz
paranoia 79 Verfolgungswahn, Paranoia
parking spot 10T Parkplatz
part, to **play a ~ in sth** 66T bei etw eine Rolle spielen
part-time 12 Teilzeit-
partially 47 teilweise, zum Teil
particular 15T spezielle/r/s
particularly, not ~ 79 nicht besonders
pass, to **gain a ~** 12 eine Prüfung bestehen
to **pass** 12 *(Prüfung)* bestehen; **~ sth** 63 etw reichen; **~ sth on** 11 etw weitergeben; **~ over sth** 32T *hier:* über etw streichen
passage, nasal ~ 32 Nasengang
path 23T Weg
patient 6 Patient/in; 55 geduldig; **high-risk ~** 75T Risikopatient; **private ~** 9 Privatpatient/in; **walk-in ~** 23 Patient/in ohne Termin; **~ records** *pl* 6 Patientenakte(n), Patientenunterlagen; **~ record file** 19 Patientenakte, Patientendaten
pay 88 Bezahlung
to **pay attention to sth** 61 auf etw achten
peanut butter 68 Erdnussbutter

peer pressure 76 Gruppendruck/-zwang
pelvic 46T Becken-; **~ examination** 46T gynäkologische Untersuchung
pen, ballpoint ~ 27 Kugelschreiber
per cent 37 Prozent
percentage 56 Anteil, Prozentsatz
perfectly 51 völlig
to **perform sth** 13 etw ausüben
perfume 11 Parfüm
period 70 Periode; **~ of time** 76 Zeitspanne
permanent 70 dauernd
permission 17 Erlaubnis
permit, work ~ 87 Arbeitserlaubnis
person, in ~ 12 persönlich
personal 29 persönlich, privat; **~ hygiene** 11 Körperpflege
personally, to **take sth ~** 55T etw persönlich nehmen
pharmaceutical 25T pharmazeutisch, Pharma-
pharmacist 21 Apotheker/in
pharmacy 22 Apotheke
to **phone in** 46T anrufen
physical 47 körperlich
physician *AE* 7 Arzt/Ärztin; **Primary Care P~ (PCP)** *AE* 7 Allgemeinarzt/-ärztin
physiotherapist 30 Physiotherapeut/-in
to **pick: ~ sth** 87 sich etw aussuchen; **~ up** 46T abholen
picky 65 wählerisch
piece of equipment 39 Gerät, Utensil
pill 52 Pille
pillow 74 Kopfkissen
pilot trial 45 Pilotversuch, Pilotprojekt
to **place** 43 platzieren
place, to **take ~** 13 stattfinden
plant 79 Pflanze
plaque 42 Ablagerung(en)
plaster 41 Pflaster
to **play a part in sth** 66T bei etw eine Rolle spielen
plenty of 33 viel(e)
plum 56 Pflaume
point, there's no ~ in doing sth 74T es hat keinen Sinn, etw zu tun
poisoning 34 Vergiftung
police station 45 Polizeiwache
Polish 61 polnisch
polite 18 höflich
politeness 14 Höflichkeit
poor 47 schlecht, dürftig
popularity 63 Beliebtheit
to **populate** 66 bevölkern
population 60 Bevölkerung
population 65 Bevölkerung
pork 57T Schwein(efleisch)
posh 63 vornehm, etepetete
to **position** 43 positionieren
position, to **be in a ~ to do sth** 22 in der Lage sein, etw zu tun
possibility 75T Möglichkeit
postcode 18 Postleitzahl
potential 11 potenziell
powder 44 Pulver
power 67 Kraft, Macht
powerful 79 stark
practical nurse, licensed ~ *AE* 80 staatlich geprüfte/r Krankenpflegehelfer/in
practice 9 Übung, Training; 9 Praxis; **general ~** 12 Allgemeinarztpraxis; **P~ makes perfect.** 86T Übung macht den Meister.
practice nurse, general ~ *BE* 80 *brit. Arzthelfer/in, die ausschließlich Behandlungsaufgaben erledigt*
practice manager 12 Praxismanager/in
to **practise** 17 üben; **~ sth** 11 etw praktizieren
practitioner, General P~ (GP) *BE* 7 Allgemeinarzt/-ärztin
pre-booked 21 im Voraus gebucht
to **prefer** 15T vorziehen, (lieber) mögen
prefrontal cortex 76 präfrontale Cortex
pregnancy 57T Schwangerschaft
pregnant 29T schwanger
prehypertension 42 Prähypertonie
preparation 44 Präparat, (Arznei-) Mittel; 86T Vorbereitung
to **prepare** 6 (sich) vorbereiten; 58 *(Essen)* kochen, zubereiten
prescreen 75T Voruntersuchung, Vorgespräch
to **prescribe** 33 verschreiben, verordnen
prescription 16 (ärztliches) Rezept, Verordnung; 44 rezeptpflichtig; **non~** 44 nicht rezeptpflichtig, rezeptfrei; **~ charge** 22 Rezeptgebühr
to **present** 37 darstellen; 45 zeigen, präsentieren
present 51T anwesend
presentation 55 Präsentation, Vortrag
presenter 70 Moderator/in; 75 Vortragende/r, Dozent/in
to **press** 73 drücken
pressure 9 Druck; **high blood ~** 42 Bluthochdruck
pretty 33 ziemlich, recht
previous 82 vorige/r/s
price 27 Preis; **total ~** 27 Gesamtpreis
primarily 65 zu(aller)erst
Primary Care Physician (PCP) *AE* 7 Allgemeinarzt/-ärztin
to **print** 26 drucken, ausdrucken
printer 26 Drucker
printout 26 Ausdruck
privacy 73 Privatsphäre
private patient 9 Privatpatient/in
probably 33 wahrscheinlich
procedure 13 Vorgehen, Verfahren(sweise)
process 13 Ablauf, Verfahren, Prozess
to **produce** 71 erstellen, herstellen
producer 79 Hersteller/in, Produzent/in
production 79 Herstellung, Produktion
professional 7 professionell; 7 beruflich; 21 Fachmann/-frau; **~ association** 83 Berufsverband
profusely, to **sweat ~** 79 stark schwitzen
program *AE* 13 Programm
programme 12 Programm *BE*; 63 (Fernseh-, Radio-)Sendung
progress 49T Fortschritt; 77 Fortgang, Fortschreiten
progressive 61 fortschreitend
prompt 85 Stichwort
prompt(ly) 17 unverzüglich, prompt
proof 79 Beweis(e)
proper(ly) 24 richtig, anständig
property 76 Eigentum
pros and cons *pl* 63 Für und Wider
to **protect** 39 schützen
to **provide** 17 bieten, liefern, zur Verfügung stellen
provider 44 Anbieter, Träger
provocative 11 provokant
psychological 65 psychologisch
psychosis 79 Psychose
pub 88 Kneipe
puberty 76 Pubertät
public 22 öffentlich, staatlich; **~ holiday** 20T (gesetzlicher) Feiertag
pulse 37 Puls; to **take sb's ~** 37 jds Puls messen
to **pump** 43 pumpen
purge 67 (kontrolliertes) Erbrechen
to **purge** 64T (kontrolliert) erbrechen
purging 64T (kontrolliertes) Erbrechen
purpose 79 Zweck
pushchair 47 Buggy *(Kinderwagen)*
pushy 65 aufdringlich, penetrant, aggressiv
to **put things right** 55T Abhilfe schaffen

Q

qualification 12 Abschluss, Qualifikation, Voraussetzung; **vocational ~** 80 Berufsabschluss;
to **qualify** 88 den Abschluss machen
quality control 79 Qualitätskontrolle
questionnaire 75T Fragebogen

quite *22* ziemlich

R

radiant *11* strahlend
radiologist *30* Radiologe/-in
radiology *72* Radiologie
to **raise** *68* erhöhen; *73* hochheben
range *79* Reihe, Spektrum; *81* Auswahl
rapeseed *BE* *57T* Raps
rash *34T* Ausschlag
rate *66* Quote; **heart ~** *37* Puls, Herzfrequenz
rather *48* eher, lieber
to **reach** *66* erreichen
to **react** *55T* reagieren
reaction *29T* Reaktion
reading *42* Wert, Messwert
ready, to **get sth ~** *39T* etw vorbereiten
reality *63* Wirklichkeit, Realität
reason *8* Grund, Begründung; **for no ~** *70* ohne Grund; to **give a ~** *8* etw begründen
reassurance *49* Beruhigung
to **reassure** *51* beruhigen
to **receive** *7* erhalten, bekommen
recently *35T* in letzter Zeit
reception *12* Empfang, Rezeption
receptionist *9* Sprechstundenhilfe
receptor *79* Rezeptor
to **recognise** *37* erkennen
to **recommend** *57T* empfehlen
recommendation *45* Empfehlung
to **record** *42* aufzeichnen, festhalten; *70* aufnehmen, *hier:* filmen
records *pl* *6* Akte(n), Unterlagen; **patient ~** *6* Patientenakte(n), Patientenunterlagen; to **keep ~** *6* Akten halten, Unterlagen führen
recovery *74T* Genesung
recreational *79* Erholungs-, Freizeit-
to **reduce** *55T* verringern
reduction *51* Rückgang
to **refer: ~ to sth** *10* sich auf etw beziehen; **~ sb to sb** *22* jdn zu jdm überweisen
reference *83* Referenz, Zeugnis; **customer ~ number** *27* Kundennummer
referral *23* Überweisung
region *76* Bereich, Region
to **register (with sb)** *7* (sich) (bei jdm) anmelden
registered nurse *80* examinierte/r Krankenschwester/-pfleger
regulation *79* Gesetzgebung, Vorschriften
related *75T* bezogen
relationship *55* Beziehung, Verhältnis
relative *12* Verwandte/r
to **relax** *7* sich entspannen
relaxed *7* locker, entspannt
relaxing *49* entspannend; **~ bath** *86T* Entspannungsbad
release, sandwich ~ *84* blockweise Freistellung
relevant to *83* relevant für, wichtig für
reliable *80* zuverlässig
to **relieve** *49T* lindern, abbauen
religious *11* religiös
to **rely on sth** *55T* auf etw angewiesen sein
to **remember** *32T* daran denken, nicht vergessen; *35T* sich (an etw) erinnern
to **remind sb of sth** *75T* jdn an etw erinnern
remote *45* fern, Fern-
to **remove** *73* entfernen, *(Kleidung)* ablegen
to **renew** *46T* erneuern
to **repair** *30* reparieren
repeat *21* Folge-
repeated *42* wiederholt
to **report** *44* melden; *63* berichten
to **represent** *83* darstellen
reputation *11* Ruf
to **require** *81* benötigen; **~ sb to do sth** *13* von jdm verlangen, etw zu tun
required *12* erforderlich, nötig
requirement *81* Anforderung; to **satisfy ~s** *12* Bedingungen erfüllen
research *68* Recherche, Nachforschungen
to **research sth** *68* etw recherchieren, Nachforschungen über etw anstellen
respect *17* Achtung, Respekt
to **respond to sth** *68* auf etw reagieren, auf etw *(Behandlung usw.)* ansprechen
response *14* Reaktion, Antwort
responsibility *83* Verantwortlichkeit, Zuständigkeit
responsible *80* verantwortungsbewusst; to **be ~ for sth** *7* für etw verantwortlich sein, für etw zuständig sein
rest *33* Ruhe; to **get some ~** *33* sich ausruhen
to **rest** *42* ruhen; **~ with sth** *83* auf etw ruhen
result *16* Ergebnis, Resultat
to **result in sth** *60* etw zur Folge haben
retail *88* Einzelhandel
retirement *81* Ruhestand
to **rid sth of sth** *63* etw von etw befreien
right, to **put things ~** *55T* Abhilfe schaffen
right away *51T* sofort
ring *17* Klingeln
to **rise** *42* steigen, ansteigen
rise *78* Anstieg, Zunahme
risk *37* Risiko, Gefahr; to **be at ~** *37* gefährdet sein; to **put sb at ~** *59* jdn einem Risiko aussetzen
to **risk** *70* riskieren, Gefahr laufen
role *12* Rolle
role-play *86* Rollenspiel
to **role-play** *19* mit verteilten Rollen spielen
roll, bread ~ *57* Brötchen
to **roll up** *35T* *(Ärmel)* hochkrempeln
roof *32T* Dach
roundabout *10T* Kreisverkehr
routine *21* (Routine-)Vorgang, Verfahren
row, in a ~ *76* nacheinander
rower *59* Ruderer/-in
royal *45* königlich
rule *11* Regel, Vorschrift
to **run: ~ sth** *45* etw leiten, etw führen; to **have ~ out** *23T* aufgebraucht sein
to **rush around** *55T* umherhetzen
rushed *49T* gehetzt

S

safety *44* Sicherheit
salad *57* Salat; **~ area** *84* Verkaufsfläche; **~ target** *82* Umsatzziel, Verkaufsziel
salmon *57* Lachs
salt *57* Salz
sample, blood ~ *6* Blutprobe; **urine ~** *46T* Urinprobe
sandal *11* Sandale
sandwich release *84* blockweise Freistellung
to **satisfy requirements** *12* Bedingungen erfüllen
saturated fats *pl* *57T* gesättigte Fettsäuren
sausage *57* (Brat-)Wurst
to **save (sb sth)** *17* (jdm etw) sparen
scale *47* Skala
scalpel *38* Skalpell
scan *30* (bildgebende) Untersuchung, Computertomographie, Scan
scared, to **be ~ of sth** *46* vor etw Angst haben
scary *46T* furchteinflößend, unheimlich
scheduling *13* Terminplanung
scheme *12* Programm, Projekt
school: comprehensive ~ *84* Gesamtschule; **vocational ~** *80* Berufsschule; to **leave ~** *31* von der Schule abgehen; **~ dinner** *63* Schulessen; **~ leaver** *12* Schulabgänger/in
science *78* (Natur-)Wissenschaft

scientific 56 wissenschaftlich
scissors *pl* 26 Schere
Scotland 45 Schottland
screen 73 Trennwand, Vorhang
to **screen sb for sth** 72 jdn auf etw hin untersuchen
screening 72 Untersuchung *(auf etw Bestimmtes)*
screwdriver 35T Schraubenzieher
to **scrub** 11 schrubben, scheuern
scrubs *pl* 11 Krankenhauskittel, OP-Kittel
seat, to **take a ~** 16T Platz nehmen
secret 79 geheim
secretarial 82T Sekretariats-
secretary, medical ~ 12 Arzthelfer/in (für Organisationsaufgaben)
section break 83 Abschnittswechsel
to **see an end to sth** 63 mit etw ein Ende machen
to **seek** 42 suchen
to **seem** 33 scheinen
seizure 79 (epileptischer) Anfall
self-care 61 Eigenfürsorge
self-control 76 Selbstbeherrschung
self-esteem 55T Selbstwertgefühl
self-exam 51T Selbstuntersuchung
self-image 67 Selbstbild
self-respect 55T Selbstachtung
senior 80 leitend, vorgesetzt, ranghöher
sensible 86T vernünftig
sensitive, to **be ~ to sth** 65 Verständnis für etw haben, verständnisvoll auf etw reagieren
serious 46T schwer, ernst, ernsthaft
seriously, to **take sth ~** 68 etw ernst nehmen
to **serve** 63 servieren
service 17 Dienstleistung, Service, Dienst
session 21 Stunde, Sitzung; **training ~** 75 Fortbildung, Lehrgang
set 79 Menge
to **set: ~ sb apart from sth** 87 sich von etw abheben; **~ out sth** 83 etw darlegen; **~ up** 45 einrichten, aufbauen
setting 13 Rahmen, Umgebung
to **settle a bill** 20T eine Rechnung bezahlen
setup 45 Aufbau, Anordnung, Einrichtung
severe 79 heftig, schlimm, schwer
sexually transmitted disease (STD) 76 sexuell übertragbare Krankheit
shape 72 Form
share 22 Teil, Anteil
shattered 20T fix und fertig, völlig erschöpft
sheet of paper 48 Blatt Papier
shirt 34T Hemd
shop assistant 82 Verkäufer/in
short-sleeved 11 kurzärmlig
shoulder 34T Schulter
shy 34T schüchtern
sick 23T krank; **sb is ~** 67 jdm ist schlecht; **~ note** 33 Krankschreibung, Attest
side effect 52 Nebenwirkung
sight 41T Anblick
to **sign** 25T unterschreiben
significant 37 bedeutend, erheblich; 78 bedeutsam, signifikant
similar (to sth) 79 (einer Sache) ähnlich
simply 55T (ganz) einfach
since 79 da, weil; 79 seit
sincerely, Yours ~ 82 *(Brief:)* Mit freundlichen Grüßen
sip 76 (kleiner) Schluck
to **sit down** 34T sich (hin)setzen
site 45 Standort
size 27 Größe; **dress ~** 70 Kleidergröße
skills *pl* 9 Fertigkeiten, Fähigkeiten
skimmed milk 58 entrahmte Milch
skin 39 Haut
skinny 70 mager, dürr
skydiving 86 Fallschirmspringen
sleeve 35T Ärmel
slim 70 schlank
to **slip** 23T ausrutschen; 35T abrutschen
to **slow sth down** 77 etw bremsen, etw verzögern
smallpox 46T Pocken
smart 81 intelligent, aufgeweckt; 86T *(Kleidung:)* schick
smear test 30 Abstrich
smell 32T Geruch
to **smell (of sth)** 48 (nach etw) riechen
to **smile** 8 lächeln
smoker 57T Raucher/in
to **sneeze** 34T niesen
snugly 43 eng, wie angegossen
so-called 76 sogenannt
soccer *AE* 66T Fußball
social care 55 Sozialfürsorge, Sozialdienste
society 72 Gesellschaft
socks *pl* 11 Socken
soft 49T leise
solid 72 fest, hart
soon, as ~ as 79 sobald; **~ enough** 64T früh genug
sore 23T wund, schlimm; **~ throat** 33 Halsschmerzen, Halsentzündung
to **sort sth out** 20T etw in Ordnung bringen
sound 43 Geräusch
to **sound** 86T klingen
south 10T Süden
spa, foot ~ 49 Fußbad
special 45 speziell, besondere/r/s; **~ offer** 27 Sonderangebot
specialist 22 Spezialist/in, Facharzt/-ärztin; Spezial-, Fach-, fachärztlich
specific 72 konkret, genau
to **specify** 77 genau angeben
spell 16 buchstabieren
spelling 16 Schreibweise
to **spend** 7 *(Zeit)* verbringen
spending 66T Ausgaben, Etat
to **spill sth** 23T etw verschütten
spinach 57T Spinat
splinter 39 Splitter
sponsored 45 gefördert
spot 34T Punkt, Fleck
to **spot** 64T erkennen
sprain 39 Verstauchung
to **spray** 79 sprühen
to **spread** 46T verbreiten
square 64 Quadrat
to **squeeze sb in** 20T *(Termin:)* jdn einschieben, jdn dazwischenschieben
staff 12 Personal, Mitarbeiter/innen; **~ appraisal** 83 Mitarbeiterbeurteilung; **~ nurse** 81 examinierte/r Krankenschwester/-pfleger
stage 42 Stufe; 45 Phase, Abschnitt
stairs *pl* 23T Treppe
to **stand** 51T stehen
standard 11 Norm
staple 27 Heftklammer
stapler 26 Hefter, Tacker
stark 78 krass
starvation 70 Hungern, Unterernährung
to **starve: ~ sb/sth of sth** 64T jdm/etw etw vorenthalten; **~ oneself** 67 hungern
state 23 Staat; staatlich; **~-provided** 14 staatlich
statement 7 Aussage, Schilderung
station 10 Bahnhof
statistics 65 Statistik(en)
status, marital ~ 83 Familienstand
to **stay awake** 86 wach bleiben
steadily 42 kontinuierlich, stetig
step 17 Schritt; to **take ~s** 65 Schritte unternehmen
sterile 7 steril
sterilization 25 Sterilisation
stethoscope 38 Stethoskop
stick, wooden ~ 51T Holzstab

stiffness *42* Steifheit
sting *39T* schmerzen, brennen
stitch *35T* Stich; to **take ~es out** *39* Fäden ziehen; to **tie off ~es** *39* Fäden vernähen
to **stitch** *39* nähen
stock levels *pl* *84* Lagerbestände
stomach *24* Magen, Bauch; **~ complaints** *pl* *52* Magenbeschwerden
stomach ache *35* Bauchschmerzen
stopover *20T* Zwischenlandung
storeroom *25* Lagerraum
straight on *10T* geradeaus
straight(away) *22* sofort
strength *83* Stärke
to **stress** *75T* betonen
stressed *37* gestresst
stressful *86T* anstrengend, stressig
stroke *79* Schlaganfall
study *12* Studium, Ausbildung; *56* Untersuchung, Studie
to **study for sth** *12* sich auf etw vorbereiten, für etw lernen
stuff, … and ~ *82T* … und so
style *11* Art, Ausführung
subject *83* (Schul-, Studien-)Fach
substance *58* Stoff, Substanz
to **succeed** *45* Erfolg haben, erfolgreich sein
success *55* Erfolg
successful(ly) *13* erfolgreich
to **suffer from sth** *48* an etw leiden
sufferer *64T* Erkrankte/r, Patient/in
sugar *57* Zucker
sugary *59* süß, zuckerhaltig
to **suggest** *22* nahelegen, andeuten
suggestion *47* Vorschlag
suitable *12* geeignet, passend
sum *26* Summe; to **do ~s** *26* rechnen
summary *45* Zusammenfassung
to **supervise** *13* beaufsichtigen, überwachen
supervisor *11* Vorgesetzte/r
supplement, dietary ~ *44* Nahrungsergänzungsmittel
supplies *pl* *7* Bedarf, Artikel, Waren; **medical ~** *9* Sanitätsartikel
support *61* Hilfe, Unterstützung; **~ group** *75T* Selbsthilfegruppe
to **suppose** *49T* annehmen, glauben
to **suppress sth** *87* etw unterdrücken
sure *10T* sicher, (na) klar
surely *66T* sicher(lich), bestimmt
surgery *BE* *7* (Arzt-)Praxis; *21* Sprechstunde, Sprechzimmer
surgical *6* chirurgisch; **~ instruments** *pl* *6* Operationsbesteck, chirurgische Instrumente
sure, to **make ~** *7* dafür sorgen; **for ~** *74T* (ganz) sicher
surname *18* Nachname
surprise, to **take sb by ~** *78* jdn erstaunen, jdn verblüffen
surprising *83* erstaunlich
suspicious *72T* verdächtig
swab *33* Abstrich; *38* Tupfer
to **swallow** *32T* schlucken
to **sweat profusely** *79* stark schwitzen
swelling *44* Schwellung, Anschwellen
swing, mood ~ *65* Stimmungsschwankung
swollen *23T* geschwollen
to **symbolize** *11* symbolisieren
symptom *30* Symptom
synthetic *79* synthetisch
to **syringe** *30* *(Ohren)* ausspülen
syringe, hypodermic ~ *38* Injektionsspritze
syrup, maple ~ *57* Ahornsirup
systolic *42* systolisch

T

table, examination ~ *73* Untersuchungsliege
tablet *33* Tablette
to **take: ~ in** *32T* *(Luft)* einatmen; **~ off** *34T* *(Kleidung)* ausziehen; *45* durchstarten, sich verbreiten; **~ action** *23* Maßnahme(n) ergreifen; **~ care of sb/sth** *22* sich um jdn/etw kümmern; *55* auf jdn/etw aufpassen, sich um jdn kümmern; **~ effect** *39T* wirken; **~ place** *13* stattfinden; **~ steps** *65* Schritte unternehmen; **~ sth personally** *55T* etw persönlich nehmen; **~ sth seriously** *68* etw ernst nehmen; **~ sb by surprise** *78* jdn erstaunen, jdn verblüffen; **~ your life** *67* sich umbringen
talk *55* Vortrag
talkative *80* gesprächig
target, sales ~ *82* Umsatzziel, Verkaufsziel
task *55T* Aufgabe
taste *32T* Geschmack
to **taste** *32T* schmecken
taxpayer *22* Steuerzahler/in
technical *83* technisch, Fach-
technology *45* Technik, Technologie
telemedicine *45* Telemedizin
temperature *24* Temperatur, Fieber; to **have a ~** *24* Fieber haben, erhöhte Temperatur haben; to **take one's ~** *33* bei jdm Fieber messen
tempered, ill-~ *55T* griesgrämig, verärgert
temping agency *82T* Zeitarbeitsfirma
temporary *82T* befristet
to **tend to do sth** *79* dazu neigen, etw zu tun
tense *47* angespannt
terrible *34T* fürchterlich
tetanus *46T* Tetanus
tetrahydrocannabinol (THC) *79* Tetrahydrocannabinol (THC)
therapy *65* Therapie
therefore *55T* daher, deshalb
thermometer *33* Thermometer
thinness *70* Schlankheit
though, even ~ *70* obwohl
thought *65* Gedanke, Überlegung
thread, needle-~ combination *38* Nadel-Faden-Kombination
throat *32* Rachen, Hals; **sore ~** *33* Halsschmerzen, Halsentzündung
thyroid *78* Schilddrüse
tidy *7* ordentlich
to **tidy** *9* aufräumen
to **tie off stitches** *39* Fäden vernähen
tight *41* eng, fest
tightness *44* Engegefühl
tiny *51T* klein
tip *71* Hinweis, Tipp
tired *33* müde
title *18* Titel, Anrede
tongue *32* Zunge
tonsillitis *33* Mandelentzündung
tonsils *pl* *33* Mandeln
tooth, teeth *32T* Zahn, Zähne
topic *13* Thema
total price *27* Gesamtpreis
tough *78* schwierig, hart
tourniquet *38* Stauschlauch, Venenstauer
toy *47* Spielzeug
trachea *32* Trachea
tract, urinary ~ *44* Harntrakt
traffic *86T* (Straßen-)Verkehr
to **train** *55* eine Ausbildung machen
trained *48* geschult, ausgebildet
trainee *32* Auszubildende/r
trainer *86* Ausbilder/in
training *12* Ausbildung; **~ session** *75* Fortbildung, Lehrgang
train station *10* Bahnhof
to **transfer** *83* übertragen
traumatic *65* traumatisch
tray *31* Schale
to **treat** *7* behandeln
treatment *14* Behandlung; **~ room** *25T* Behandlungsraum

trial *45* Test, Versuch; **pilot ~** *45* Pilotversuch, Pilotprojekt
trimmed fingernails *pl* *11* kurze Fingernägel
to **triple** *66* sich verdreifachen
trouble *33* Schwierigkeit(en), Problem(e)
truly *87* wirklich, wahrhaftig
trust *55T* Vertrauen
to **trust** *49T* vertrauen
truth *48* Wahrheit
to **try** *7* versuchen
tube *32T* Röhre
tummy *70* Bauch
tumour *74T* Geschwulst, Tumor
turn, to **take (it in) ~s in doing sth** *35* etw abwechselnd tun
to **turn** *74T* (sich) wenden; **~ to sth** *65* sich einer Sache zuwenden; **~ sth down** *76* etw ablehnen; **~ left/right** *10T* links/rechts abbiegen
TV show *63* Fernsehsendung, -serie
tweezers *pl* *38* Pinzette
twice *52* zweimal
type *59* Typ
typical *6* typisch
typically *13* normalerweise, üblicherweise

U

ultrasound *73* Ultraschall
umbrella stand *20T* Schirmständer
unable *66* unfähig
unattractive *70* unattraktiv
uncomfortable, to **feel ~** *47* sich unwohl fühlen
uncontrolled *65* unkontrolliert
under-age *76* minderjährig, bei/von Minderjährigen
underground *10* U-Bahn
underground station *10T* U-Bahn-Station
understanding *55T* Verständnis
underweight *60* untergewichtig
to **undress** *47* sich ausziehen
undressed, to **get ~** *73* sich ausziehen
unfortunately *68* leider
unfriendly *48* unfreundlich
unhealthy *60* ungesund
uniform *11* Arbeitskleidung
unimportant *72* unwichtig, unbedeutend
unit *68* Einheit, Maßeinheit; *72* Gerät
university *80* Universität
unless *52* wenn nicht
unnatural(ly) *71* unnatürlich
unsuitable *11* ungeeignet, unpassend
unsweetened *57T* ungesüßt
until *43* bis
up to date *7* auf dem neuesten Stand, aktuell
upper *42* obere/r/s
upper clothing *73* Oberbekleidung
upset *7* aufgebracht, verstört
urgency *17* Dringlichkeit
urgent *14* dringend
urinary tract *44* Harntrakt
urine sample *46T* Urinprobe
Uruguayan *70* aus Uruguay
usage *68* Verbrauch
usually *13* normalerweise, gewöhnlich
use, to **make ~ of sth** *82T* etw nutzen, sich etw zunutze machen
user, drug ~ *79* Drogenabhängige/r

V

vaccination *46T* Impfung, Schutzimpfung
valid *87* gültig
value *42* Wert
valve *43* Ventil
vascular *42* Gefäß-
vegetable oil *57T* Pflanzenöl
vegetables *pl* *57* Gemüse
verbal *81* mündlich
versatile *83* vielseitig
victory *63* Sieg
to **video** *20T* (auf Video) aufnehmen
video conferencing *45* Videokonferenz(schaltung)
view *37* Ansicht
viewer *63* Zuschauer/in
vision, blurred ~ *52* verschwommenes Sehen
visit, home ~ *23T* Hausbesuch
vitamin *57T* Vitamin
vocational course *80* Berufsbildungskurs
vocational qualification *80* Berufsabschluss
vocational school *80* Berufsschule
to **volunteer** *45* sich (freiwillig) zur Verfügung stellen; *87* ehrenamtlich arbeiten
to **vomit** *34T* sich erbrechen
vomiting *79* Erbrechen

W

waiting room *8* Wartezimmer
to **walk into sth** *19* in etw (herein) kommen
walk-in patient *23* Patient/in ohne Termin
warmth *55T* Wärme
to **warn** *78* warnen, hinweisen
warning signal *37* Warnsignal
wax *30* Ohrenschmalz
way, in no ~ *79* in keiner Weise; to **get in the ~ of sth** *43* einer Sache im Wege sein
weakness *55T* Schwäche
wedding ring *24* Ehering
to **weigh** *65* abwiegen, wiegen
weight *59* Gewicht; to **lose ~** *59* abnehmen; **body ~** *64T* Körpergewicht; **~ loss** *64T* Gewichtsverlust, -abnahme
welcome, You're ~. *14* Bitte. Gern geschehen.
well, as ~ *34T* auch, und; **as ~ as** *82* ebenso wie
well-cooked *78* *(Fleisch:)* durchgebraten
well-organized *80* gut organisiert
wheel *76* Rad, *hier:* Lenkrad, Steuer
wheelchair *47* Rollstuhl
whether *22* ob
whole *45* ganz
whole milk *68* Vollmilch
wide *33* weit
windpipe *32* Luftröhre
within *12* in, innerhalb
wooden stick *51T* Holzstab
to **work: ~ sth out** *27* etw ausrechnen
work: ~ experience *12* Berufs-/Arbeitserfahrung; **~ permit** *87* Arbeitserlaubnis; **~ routine** *81* Arbeitsablauf
work-based assignment *12* praktische Prüfungsaufgabe
workman *20T* Handwerker
workplace *6* Arbeitsplatz
World Health Organization (WHO) *70* Weltgesundheitsorganisation
worldwide *60* weltweit
worried *47* besorgt, beunruhigt
to **worry about sth** *47* sich um etw Sorgen machen
wound *39* Wunde
writing, in ~ *81* schriftlich
written *12* schriftlich

XY

X-rays *pl* *9* Röntgenstrahlen; to **take ~** *9* röntgen
yet, not … ~ *10T* noch nicht
yoghurt *57T* Joghurt
you may find *7* es kann sein, es kann vorkommen
You're welcome. *14* Bitte. Gern geschehen.
Yours sincerely *82* *(Brief:)* Mit freundlichen Grüßen

IV Irregular Verbs

be – was/were – been	sein
beat – beat – beaten	schlagen, besiegen
become – became – become	werden
begin – began – begun	anfangen, beginnen
break – broke – broken	brechen
bring – brought – brought	bringen
build – built – built	bauen
burn – burnt/burned – burnt/burned	(ver)brennen
buy – bought – bought	kaufen
catch – caught – caught	fangen
choose – chose – chosen	wählen
come – came – come	kommen
cost – cost – cost	kosten
cut – cut – cut	schneiden
deal (with) – dealt (with) – dealt (with)	sich kümmern um, umgehen mit
do – did – done	tun, machen
draw – drew – drawn	zeichnen
dream – dreamt/dreamed – dreamt/dreamed	träumen
drink – drank – drunk	trinken
drive – drove – driven	fahren
eat – ate – eaten	essen
fall – fell – fallen	fallen
feed – fed – fed	füttern, ernähren
feel – felt – felt	(sich) fühlen, empfinden
fight – fought – fought	kämpfen
find – found – found	finden
fit – fit/fitted – fit/fitted	passen
fly – flew – flown	fliegen
forget – forgot – forgotten	vergessen
get – got – got (*AE* gotten)	bekommen
give – gave – given	geben
go – went – gone	gehen, fahren
grow – grew – grown	wachsen
hang – hung – hung	hängen
have – had – had	haben
hear – heard – heard	hören
hide – hid – hidden	(sich) verstecken
hit – hit – hit	schlagen
hold – held – held	halten, festhalten
hurt – hurt – hurt	verletzen, wehtun
keep – kept – kept	behalten
know – knew – known	kennen, wissen
lay – laid – laid	legen
lead – led – led	führen
learn – learnt/learned – learnt/learned	lernen
leave – left – left	abfahren, verlassen, weggehen
let – let – let	lassen
lie – lay – lain	liegen
light – lit – lit	anzünden, beleuchten, anmachen
lose – lost – lost	verlieren
make – made – made	machen
mean – meant – meant	meinen, bedeuten
meet – met – met	treffen
pay – paid – paid	bezahlen
put – put – put	setzen, stellen, legen
read – read – read	lesen
ride – rode – ridden	reiten, fahren
ring – rang – rung	klingeln, anrufen
rise – rose – risen	(an)steigen
run – ran – run	laufen, rennen
say – said – said	sagen
see – saw – seen	sehen
sell – sold – sold	verkaufen
send – sent – sent	senden, schicken
set – set – set	setzen, stellen
shake – shook – shaken	schütteln
show – showed – shown	zeigen
shut – shut – shut	schließen
sing – sang – sung	singen
sit – sat – sat	sitzen
sleep – slept – slept	schlafen
smell – smelt/smelled – smelt/smelled	riechen
speak – spoke – spoken	sprechen
spell – spelt/spelled – spelt/spelled	buchstabieren
spend – spent – spent	ausgeben, verbringen
stand – stood – stood	stehen
steal – stole – stolen	stehlen
stick – stuck – stuck	kleben
swim – swam – swum	schwimmen
take – took – taken	nehmen
teach – taught – taught	unterrichten, beibringen
tell – told – told	sagen, erzählen
think – thought – thought	denken
throw – threw – thrown	werfen
understand – understood – understood	verstehen
wake – woke – woken	wecken
wear – wore – worn	tragen (Kleidung)
win – won – won	gewinnen
write – wrote – written	schreiben

Abbildungsverzeichnis

Cartoonstock: 8 Cartoonstock/Fran; 60 Cartoonstock/Aaron Bacall; 86 Cartoonstock/Aaron Bacall; 55 un. Cartoonstock/Mark Godfrey.

Shutterstock: 6 A Lisa F. Young; 6 B Rob Bouwman; 6 C Giovanni G; 6 D Africa Studio; 6 E Monkey Business Images; 6 F bikeriderlondon; 14 ESB Professional; 27 Minerva Studio; 33 Image Point Fr; 23B Image Point Fr; 23 C Family Business; 23 D ZoneFatal; 30 A Nadino; 30 B Hans Kim; 30 C wavebreakmedia; 30 D Ollyy; 30 E; T-Design; 30 F Karyna Che; 34 B sheff; 34 D Dean Drobot; 34 E Stephanie Frey; 46 (1) sonya etchison; 46 (2) Tiplyashina Evgeniya; 46 (3) goodluz; 46 (4) szefei; 46 (5) iofoto; 47 LOGVINYUK YULIIA; 48 hxdbzxy; 49 VGstockstudio; 50 (2) Tamara83; 50 (4) Sidarta; 50 (6) You can more; 56 (1) Ekaterina Bratova; 56 (2) Evan Lorne; 56 (4) Evan Lorne; 56 (5) Robyn Mackenzie; 59 Andrey_Popov; 64 ob. Hugo Felix; 65 Vgstockstudio; 71 Debby Wong; 74 (1) edwardolive; 74 (2) Fotoluminate LLC; 74 (3) Tyler Olson; 74 (4) Suzi44; 74 (5) WhiteJack; 80 A Andrey_Popov; 80 B goodluz; 82 (2) wavebreakmedia; 82 (3) S_L; 82 (4) Olena Zaskochenko; 88 IR Stone.

Fotolia: Cover gamjai; 12 contrastwerkstatt; 18 auremar; 20 Africa Studio; 22 © Robert Kneschke; 23 A www.foto-und-mehr.de; 23 E haveseen; 29 Andreas Keudel © ISO K° - photography; 34 A Andrey Kiselev; 34 C Alen-D; 45 Rocketclips inc; 50 (1) Tyler Olson; 50 (5) Guido Grochowski; 50 (7) Winfried Eckl; 51 Zsolnai Gergely; 52 Peter Atkins; 53 (3) Sebastian Luenenstrass; 55 ob. contrastwerkstatt; 61 Dan Race; 64 un. tortoon; 67 Photographee.eu; 72 © Robert Kneschke; 77 © 2012 Markus W. Lambrecht; 80 C contrastwerkstatt; 82 (1) denisismagilov.

Imagetrust: 31 ob. Klaus Rose; **plainpicture:** 31 un.; interTOPICS/ddp images: 63; **OKAPIA:** 50 (3) Jochen Tack/imageBROKER/OKAPIA.

Textverzeichnis

S. 44 text: Cranberry is used for, source: http://www.drugs.com/cdi/cranberry.html
S. 69 text: Orthorexie: Wenn gesundes Essen zwanghaft wird, source: http://www.abendblatt.de/nachrichten/article206863583/Orthorexie-Wenn-gesundes-Essen-zwanghaft-wird.html; author: Dpa/Hamburger Abendblatt
S. 78 text: Dealing With Chronic Illnesses and Depression, source: http://www.webmd.com/depression/guide/chronic-illnesses-depression?page=2#2; author: Joseph Goldberg, MD/WebMD LLC
S. 87 text: Gain knowledge and work experience in the UK, source: http://www.internship-uk.com, author: Internship UK, London
S. 78 text: Cancer Cases In Children Leap By 40% In 16 Years, source: http://news.sky.com/story/cancer-cases-in-children-up-by-40-10564534, author: Katie Spencer/Sky News UK

Danksagung

Many thanks go to Dr Catherine Tooley MbChb, MRCPCH, MRCGP for her support, input and generosity with her time.